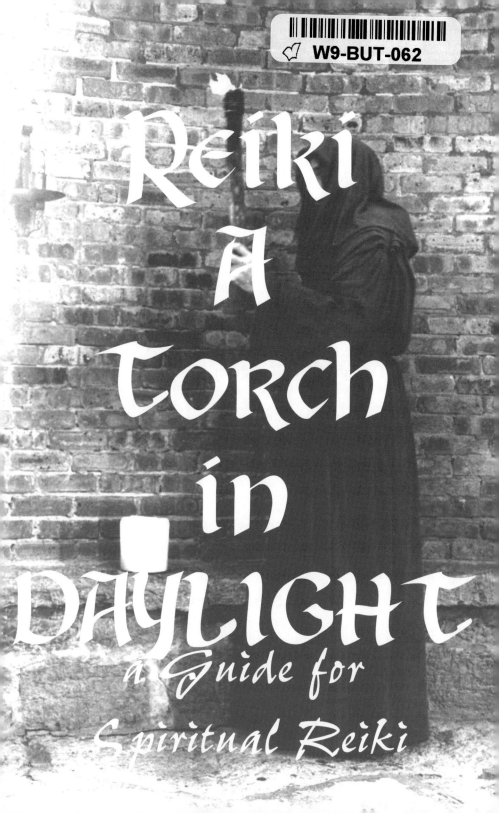

Reiki A Torch in DAYLIGHT

a Guide for

Spiritual Reiki

Reiki, A Torch In Daylight

Library of Congress Cataloging-in-Publication Data
Mitchell, Karyn
Reiki, A Torch In Daylight
ISBN 0-9640822-1-7
1. Healing 2. Alternative Medicine
94-075679

Cover Photo by Shauna Angelblue
Cover Design by Bob Tentinger

Mind Rivers Publications
603 Geneva Road, St. Charles, IL 60174
815-732-7150

Printed in the United States of America

7 8 9 10

Reiki A Torch in Daylight

by Karyn Mitchell N.D., Ph.D.

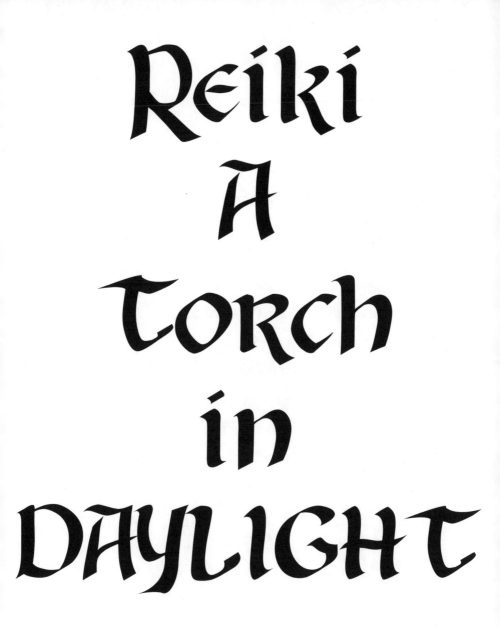

Free your mind. Free your heart.
Free your spirit.
As you hold this glorious gift in
the palm of each hand,
You are the creator of your own
universe, you are Chiron,
The once wounded healer, now
transformed and limitless.
It is so. It has been ordained by
you, the creator-healer.
The dreamer of perfection incar-
nate living in harmony.
You who reflect in your radiant,
loving, healing heart,
The lifeblood of the star-filled
Cosmos: of All That Is...
You, the Divine Gift, reflect
the wondrous image
        of the
            beautiful
                moon.

                        KM

TABLE OF CONTENTS

TABLE OF CONTENTS *(Continued)*

霊気 *Reiki*
USUI SHIKI RYOHO

Reiki Principles
Just for today
 Do not anger
Just for today
 Do not worry
Honor your parents
 teachers and elders
Earn your living honestly
Show gratitude
 to every living thing

Reiki Path Empowerment

Reiki is one of the greatest gifts that you can give yourself and share with others. Why do I say this? Because Reiki is all about love, balance, and empowerment.

BALANCE is the Eastern concept that translates into promoting body harmony; preventative medicine, if you will. The practitioner who daily meditates, utilizing a form of self healing, will find that diseases are no longer a fact of life. The Emotional, Mental, Spiritual, and Physical bodies are maintained in good health and a feeling of well-being results.

EMPOWERMENT comes as a direct result of balance and harmony. The individual who knows what the body, mind, spirit, and emotions need is aware that they also have direct control over life. You no longer have to give your power away to others to help you achieve health, happiness, and well-being. This brings in a feeling of power, a sense of wholeness that springs from joy. A person who lives in joy lives in a state of love and power over outside influences. This person has found the way, the path to happiness. This is the REIKI PATH.

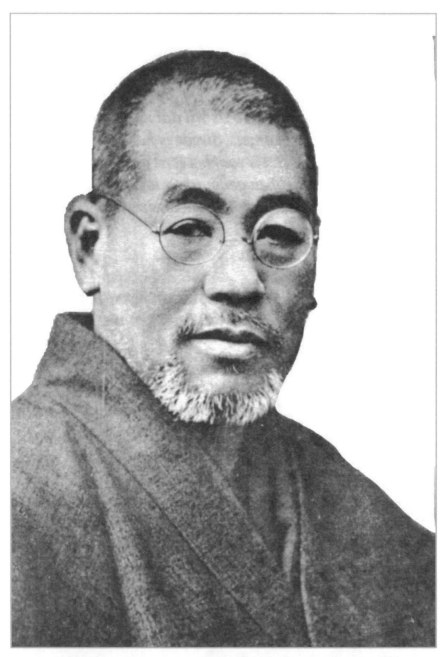

Master Mikao Usui

A Torch in Daylight by Reiki Master Karyn K. Mitchell

A TORCH IN DAYLIGHT
PURPOSE & INTENTION

A Torch In Daylight is separated into sections or levels of study, from First Degree Reiki to Reiki Master-Teacher. My hope is that it can be utilized as a teaching and learning tool for structured classes, and also facilitate a clearer understanding concerning the healing modality of Reiki.

It was a goal of mine to represent Reiki in this book in as pure a form as I personally could, holding to the Eastern traditions of healing wherever possible. Reiki blends so well with so many other healing methods that it has led to many combined therapy approaches. For example: Reiki and Crystal and Stone Healing, Reiki and Massage Therapy (Shiatsu, Reflexology, Orthobiotomy, Sacral Cranial, Rolfing), Reiki and Touch For Health, Reiki and Hypnotherapy, and even Reiki and Esoteric and Christian Doctrines. I embrace all of these, and work with a combined therapy approach often. But this is not just Reiki, it is Reiki and something else. In my next book, *Reiki: Beyond The Usui System,* I will share with you some of these combined approaches that I find most useful.

The symbols for Reiki are not to be found in this book, as they are useful as a healing tool only for those individuals who have been empowered to use them. In traditional Reiki, we hold these symbols sacred (which means secret), so if you are called to learn Reiki, your Master will share these symbols with you at the appropriate time. This book is based upon Traditional Reiki.

I would like to thank Steve Mitchell, my dear husband, and Robert Tentinger, a dear friend, two men whose technical and spiritual help have made this book a physical reality. They have worked as hard on this as I have, and I greatly appreciate and acknowledge their help. I also appreciate the artistic perception of photographer, Shauna AngelBlue, and the encouragement of all of my Reiki friends and students through the years.

I humbly dedicate this book to Master Usui, whose desire to connect the spirit with the physical has had a profound effect of healing and love on my life. May all who were Reiki before us and all who will be Reiki after us guide your spirit in love and light.

Know you're never alone on the Reiki Healing Path

A Blessing from the Tibetan Masters

A Blessing from Master Mikao Usui

A Blessing from Master Karyn Mitchell

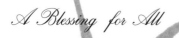

A Blessing for You

A Blessing for All

A Torch in Daylight by Reiki Master Karyn K. Mitchell

Description of Classes
Reiki Path Empowerment
Reiki 1

The student is introduced to a simple meditation technique in order to prepare for the Reiki I initiation. When the student is ready, there is a transfer of energy that opens you up to a universal energy we call Reiki (Ray-Key). You then become a facilitator for channeling healing energy. Hand positions for a table treatment, chair and quick treatment, self treatment, and the Reiki Boost are introduced, as well as the chakra system, visualization, history, sweeping the aura, closing, Reiki Precepts and Principles, and ethics. It starts a twenty-one day cleansing cycle of the seven major chakras.

霊

気

Reiki

Reiki 11

Introduces the symbols that are used for Absentia healing as well as symbols to work with such issues such as past-life, karmic, mental healing, and emotional healing. You will learn to send Reiki to other places at other times to yourself and others. The energy transfer further opens you to the Reiki energy. Advanced healing techniques are shared. It also starts a twenty-one day cleansing cycle of the seven major chakras.

Reiki 111

Completely opens you to the Reiki energy. It also starts another twenty-one day cleansing cycle of the seven chakras. You receive the highest attunements as well as instruction and practice in using the symbols in the complete Usui system. You are also introduced to the water ceremony, Vertical Treatments, 18 Beyond the Usui System Symbols, Mental Healing, Nine Nurturing Four Ki Bodies, Tonglen, and other meditations.

Reiki Master Teacher Training and Certification

Is also available for those who desire to empower others with the complete system of holistic healing and personal development. The Master/Teacher course is linked with much fulfillment and growth as well as having a special blessing of its own. You learn to teach the Usui Shiki Ryoho.

THE FIRST DEGREE CLASS
in Reiki

Reiki Only Works For Good

Reiki empowerment comes through a series of initiations that increase power at each level or "degree." It is much like a three-way light bulb. The first light transmission is dimmer than the second, and the third transmission is the brightest. In our particular tradition of Reiki, there are three levels of empowerment. There are other traditions that have more initiations, but all paths merge at the same level of Reiki Master energy.

The followers of Master Usui would receive initiations at regular intervals, when they were deemed prepared to go on. In order now to insure that the energies are increased at a level that can be more easily integrated, we recommend the system of a twenty-one day waiting period between each of the three empowerment initiations. This allows for the cleansing process to clear each of the seven axis chakras three times. It also promotes self-healing, and maximum integration of positive energies.

Once you have been initiated into Reiki, the empowerment for healing yourself and others is available to you for the rest of your life. It cannot be taken away from you, but you can choose not to use this gift. It is a matter of your will, as Reiki will never transgress the will of any person. It can be used only for good, never for less than what we call Divine Order. Just because you or your ego hold an outcome in mind, if it is not ordained by the higher self of the individual, it will not be so. We are merely what we call channels in Reiki for the higher energies, so we must transcend the ego, we must go beyond performance expectations. It is my hope that you will be patient and learn to trust and honor Reiki's powerful healing process.

Occasionally I will meet a person who feels that they are performing healings without the need or benefit of empowerment initiations. What I say to them is, "good for you!" I also explain that I have been doing similar energy work since I was eleven, working mostly with animals in my earlier years. It is all a matter of faith, is it not? And faith can move mountains. However, we must remember that just because WE wish someone to be well, it doesn't always happen. And then we tend to lose faith in what we perceive is our ability to heal. Reiki gives us a complete system, a solid base for healing. Reiki is an ancient system. Some believe that it stems from Atlantean times, if you believe, as I do, that there was an Atlantis. It is at least traced back to Sutra documents 2,500 years old.

Western Allopathic Medicine, by comparison, is still in its infant stages at 200 years old. Beyond being a system, Reiki empowers you more as your energy is at least squared at each consecutive level of initiation. What I have found to be generally true is that all people have some level of healing power. The amount may be due, to some extent, to what they feel is possible for them. However, the energy level generally does not match Reiki Level I energies. This is certainly not an attempt on my part to take away anyone's power; I am merely explaining from my own experience how or why Reiki can be beneficial even to those who have already been doing divine healing work.

I will relate to you what I teach in Reiki Level I, and how I structure this class. We teach Reiki as a Spiritual Healing Art, as that is traditional Reiki.

◆ REIKI PRINCIPLES AND PRECEPTS. AN EXPLANATION AND ENDORSEMENT OF THE REIKI PRINCIPLES AND PRECEPTS.

◆ HISTORY OF REIKI, HOW REIKI WORKS. (Short Break)

◆ DISCUSSION OF THE TWENTY-ONE DAY CLEARING (HEALING) CYCLE.

◆ DEMONSTRATION OF THE INITIATION PROCESS.

◆ GUIDED MEDITATION.

◆ INITIATION CEREMONY. (ATTUNEMENT)

◆ JOINING OF ENERGIES IN A CIRCLE. BREAK OR LUNCH.

◆ REIKI BOOST, SELF HEALING, QUICK TREATMENT, TABLE WORK.

◆ ASSIGNMENTS: DREAM AND HEALING JOURNAL. DAILY SELF TREATMENTS. MUST TRY ONE TABLE TREATMENT WITH ANOTHER BEING.

◆ CLOSING CIRCLE. SHARING "BE WELL" HUGS.

It is important to come to Reiki Classes well rested, as there is much to integrate into the physical, mental, emotional and spiritual bodies. Some leave class feeling full of energy, while others may feel mentally stressed. It is always an honor to serve as a teacher to those whose path has led to Reiki. Enjoy the energy, engage in Self Treatment daily, and be well.

REIKI PRINCIPLES & PRECEPTS

In Reiki Level One, the first exercise that we do is to read, discuss and then affirm the five Reiki Principles and the two Spiritual Precepts. I want to be certain that each student understands on some level what is expected of a person who wishes to integrate Reiki into their everyday life.

HISTORY OF THE SPIRITUAL PRECEPTS

It is important to comprehend the birth of these Precepts. When Master Usui worked in the Beggar's Quarters, in the slums of Kyoto, he offered his healings in exchange for a place to sleep there and three bowls of rice a day. However, he noticed after a certain length of time that some of those whom he had healed returned to the slums. When he asked them why they had returned, they told him that it was easier to stay as they were, beggars in the slums, than it was to earn a living. He had failed in his healing work on some level, he felt. He realized that the beggars did not value their healing. After intense meditation, he realized that he had healed the physical bodies of the beggars, but not the spiritual. There has to be a raising of consciousness for true healing to begin: all healing begins on the spiritual level. He also discovered that there needed to be an exchange of energy for the person to value the energy. Thus the two Spiritual Precepts of Reiki were born from the meditation of Master Mikao (Mick-kow) Usui (Ou-suey).

TEST OF TIME: *Time and Emotions*

The Five Reiki Principles are just as applicable today as they were in Master Usui's day. Some of the ways in class that we discuss the various Principles are as follows:

We begin with the first three words, "JUST FOR TODAY..." This limits the focus, the expanse of time to the present, forcing us to live in the cosmic "now" This removes all stress related barriers that can overload the consciousness. For example, •••"Just for today, do not anger," means that anger, which is generally tied to responses in the past, is no longer serving you at this present time. If you choose to act in your truth rather than react to some outside force or person, then it is not necessary to have anger in your life. Believe it or not, anger is a conscious choice related to some event in your past. You can choose not to be angry just for today...

In just the same way, you can choose not to worry. Worry is related to your response to a probable event in the future, rather than a response based on the past (anger). Your frame of reference shifts to reacting on the basis of what if; a future event that is not only unrealized, but probably will never be. By centering in the now and focusing on what is real, there is no need for worry. Worrying is useless for someone who lives fully in the moment. The now is the reality. •••"Just for today, do not worry."

•••"Honor your parents, teachers, and elders" (also your neighbors and friends). I believe that the intention of "honor" is to show respect in this case. I would like for you to reflect for just a moment about conscious choice. We choose our parents, before we are born; we choose our teachers, our elders and our friends. In this light then, for us not to honor or respect on some level what we have chosen, is to negate our opportunity for growth. It creates bitterness when we condemn rather than praise. We need to honor those who have helped us to incarnate and grow spiritually. Honor your parents for the gift of life even if you have come from a challenged childhood. Also remember that not all teachers are human.

•••"Earn your living honestly" is much the same. We must respect the job that we have chosen for ourselves, and honor ourselves by only doing our best to create a feeling of satisfaction in that work. All work is valuable to the extent that we value it. I truly believe that there are jobs that we should not perform; ones that would be dishonoring to the self. These should be avoided, and you must trust that the work that you have chosen is honorable and important. If it is not, then you should consider finding work that you can do honestly and feel good about doing.

As part of the Universal Life Force, you begin to feel more and more connected to ALL THAT IS. As your consciousness is raised, you know that every living thing is a part of you and you are a part of it. It is a natural evolution to •••"Show gratitude to every living thing," and know that by doing so, you are paying homage and respect to the Divine energy in all life.

Do not surrender your personal power to anger, fear, or worry. Honor yourself by honoring other humans and all of life. Peace exists in that love.

2500+ Years Ago	Sanscrit Sutras Tibetan Monks Enlightened Masters	
1890's Master Mikao Usui	1900's Dr. Chujiro Hayashi	1939 Master Hawayo Takata

→ 22 Masters

History of Reiki Masters

Master Mikao Usui

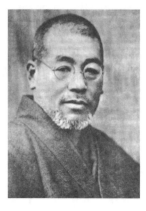

With current knowledge, we are unable to trace the true human beginnings of what we now call the healing art of "Reiki."

However, one man, Master Mikao Usui, is credited with re-discovering the process of initiation into the spiritual path of the Reiki energy. It is believed that Master Usui was born in 1865 and made his transition in 1926. There are two major historical accounts concerning Master Mikao Usui. One states that he was a Buddhist monk in Kyoto, Japan, who followed a twenty-eight year quest to rediscover how the Buddha had healed through compassion. Another account states that he was the dean of a small Christian university in Kyoto. He resigned his job at this school in order to rediscover how Jesus healed. One unsubstantiated story links Master Usui to the University of Chicago.

Both accounts merge at the Sutra studies. In Japan, Master Usui studied the Japanese Lotus Sutras (ancient teachings), the Chinese Sutras, and then, finally, the Sanskrit Sutras of Tibet. The Tibetan scrolls revealed information concerning St. Isa, which several scholars relate as the physical incarnation of Master Jesus. While Usui had the technical, mental information that he needed concerning healing, he lacked the physical and spiritual empowerment process that he needed to be able to heal. This led him to his spiritual pilgrimage on sacred Mount Kuri Yama. There he fasted and meditated for twenty-one days. He set twenty-one stones before him, as a way to count the days, and as he threw the last one away, he was struck by a powerful light in the middle of the forehead. Out of the rainbow of color that he envisioned, came bubbles of white, blue, purple, and gold. Each individual color contained the keys or symbols essential to Reiki. A voice then said to him, "These are the keys to healing; learn them, do not forget them, and do not allow them to be lost." Our particular tradition utilizes these symbols and colors in the healing and initiation process.

Master Usui returned to Kyoto where he was instructed to go to the beggar's quarters to do healing work. There he worked for seven years. He noticed that many that he had healed eventually returned to the beggar's quarters simply because they wished to escape responsibility. Again in meditation, Master Usui was given further guidance that concerned the healing of the spirit and the responsibility of the healee in the healing process. He was, at that time, given the five spiritual principles of Reiki to balance the prior physical aspect of his healing work. In our research, we believe that Master Mikao Usui was not only married, but had two children. He served as a Monk in the Japanese Buddhist tradition.

As a Master, Mikao Usui gathered a following of sixteen Masters. Before his transition, he asked one of his students, Dr. Chujiro Hayashi, a retired naval officer, to preserve the Reiki teachings, to carry the Reiki Torch.

Dr. Chujiro Hayashi

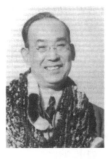

Dr. Chujiro Hayashi founded the first Reiki clinic in Tokyo, Japan in the early 1900's. There he trained thirteen masters. He was a powerful mystic and was able to foresee the future. Because he was aware that he, as well as many of his trained Masters, could be called into active service for World War II, he decided to initiate two women in order to insure that the Reiki tradition would not be lost. One woman, his wife, a Japanese national, told him that she did not desire to teach Reiki. The other, Hawayo Takata, a Japanese woman from the island of Hawaii, preserved the Reiki tradition. Hayashi trained Takata in the Reiki tradition. Before creating his own transition, in order to save many lives and maintain the spiritual principles of Reiki, he initiated Takata into the Reiki mastership. It was reported that Takata and Mrs. Hayashi were the only two Reiki masters to survive the war.

Master Hawayo Takata

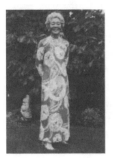

Hawayo Takata was healed in Hayashi's Reiki clinic while visiting her parents in Japan. She asked to learn Reiki in exchange for a year of work in the clinic for Dr. Hayashi. Years after her return to Hawaii, the spirit of Hayashi asked for her to return to Japan for her initiation into the mastership. Her faith preserved the Reiki tradition for all of us who *Wish to Hold the Gift of Reiki in Our Hands.* This is a dedication from the Reiki Blue Book). In the 1970's, Takata began to train others to be Reiki Masters, and by the time of her transition in December of 1980, she had trained twenty-two Reiki Master Teachers. She Westernized and Christianized the practice of Reiki.

Today there are different philosophies concerning a Reiki hierarchy. Many Reiki people recognize the granddaughter of Takata, Phyllis Lei Furumoto, as the Grand Master of Reiki. The AIRA, American Reiki Association, recognizes Barbara Weber Ray as Grand Master. Mary McFadyen, one of the twenty-two masters of Takata recognizes all Reiki Masters as equal. So do I, but with great love and gratitude for all who came before us and all who will come after us. In the Reiki tradition, as we honor the energy, we are all one.

A TORCH IN DAYLIGHT:
A BOLD STATEMENT
WITHOUT WORDS
The Grand Masters of Reiki and Their Personal Philosophies

A torch in daylight? What does that mean? Why would one need a brighter light in daytime? Master Mikao Usui pilgrimaged through many small, Japanese towns in the early 1900's, in broad daylight with a fiery, burning torch. Usui was making a bold statement without words. The torch was much more than just a device to attract attention. The torch was the way that Master Usui chose to illuminate others...to raise their conscious-ness for Reiki. While the visual brightness of the torch created curious onlookers, by FOCUSING ON THE LIGHT, those same onlookers, if they were spiritually ready, would hear, feel, and sense the TRUTH about life, about healing, about Reiki. Usui would then only hold their pulse points, and, if it was desired, if they were ready to let go of their dis-ease, they would then be healed. That is how a man named Chujiro Hayashi was introduced to Master Mikao Usui, through the unspoken message of the flaming Torch.

In the early days after his own illumination, Master Usui journeyed to the beggar's quarters in Kyoto to perform healing miracles. It must have seemed a personal defeat, at first, when the beggars in Kyoto returned to the Beggar's Quarters a year or so after their healing. This precious gift of healing, a gift from the life force itself, why did they not value and honor it? Meditation led Master Usui to the revelation of the two major precepts of Reiki. The First Precept: The person being healed had to have the desire for change, the desire to be well. The Second Precept was that there had to be an exchange of energy, a payment for Reiki Healing in order for the person being healed to honor and accept the true healing.

I found it interesting that Master Usui, after leaving the Beggar's Quar-ters in Kyoto, would wander the city streets with a lit torch in broad daylight in order to attract attention to his message. This message quite simply was that he could lead people to healing by illuminating their souls, thus raising their consciousness and vibration. Part of this philosophy derived from Buddhism, from the Sutras, or ancient teachings, that is, that the spirit must be healed first before the physical. Spirit first, then the physical. After later sharing a spiritually illuminating lecture, Master Usui would hold the pulse points of a person's hand in order to share his Reiki Healing Energy. Master Usui dedicated many years of his life to discover the way that Gautama Buddha or Jesus Christ healed those who were dis-eased. His desire was not to make himself rich with his discovery, but to help human-kind, to ease suffering and to create ease out of dis-ease.

So, in considering the energy exchange or money involved in Reiki healings, we go forward to Master Hayashi's Clinic, which was located near the Imperial Palace in Tokyo. It was a small clinic with eight tables and sixteen practitioners working at one time. Master Hayashi brought Reiki off the streets and into a professional clinic situation. When Master Hayashi taught practitioners how to perform Reiki on a client, he taught a series of four hand placements on the head, four on the front of the body, and four hand placements on the back. Other hand placements were added as needed by the body being treated. The head and trunk of the body were the focus. This is how Master Takata was taught to do Reiki.

Hawayo Takata noticed when she was a practitioner in Master Hayashi's clinic, that it was upper class or wealthy individuals who were treated with Reiki. Why, she wondered, were there not more poor people seeking treatment? She implied that perhaps Master Hayashi did not wish to treat those without a great deal of money. Not so, Master Hayashi indicated. The poor did not value Reiki, just as they did not value the less expensive medical doctors in their villages. They only trusted the doctors in the cities who charged more money for their services. The poor did not value Reiki. It took a certain level of consciousness in order to be able to understand the value of healing with the Universal Life Force Energy. This seems like a rather cruel judgment, but not one that Master Hayashi was making. It was the decision of the individual that created the space for healing. The poor people of Tokyo did not believe that Reiki could heal them. They (as do some today) did not believe that healing could take place without cutting open the body and shedding blood. Their belief system did not allow for the simplicity of the Natural Healing System called Ryoho. It seems primitive to imagine that one must suffer more pain and let more blood before healing can take place, but that is the way that many, especially in the Western Culture, still believe. Master Hayashi comprehended this belief system and did not try to impose his method of healing upon those who were not spiritually ready to accept it. We do not impose.

I am not sure what the Great Masters charged their clients for Reiki Healings. I am not sure what price Chujiro Hayashi, or any of Usui's other fifteen Masters, paid Master Usui for teaching them Reiki. We are aware, however, that Master Takata devoted an entire year of her life working in Hayashi's Clinic in order to learn the Healing Art of Reiki. How many of us today would be willing to make such a commitment? Knowing what I do now of the incredible power of Reiki, I can say that I believe I would. It was part of Takata's belief, her philosophy, that in order to be a Reiki Master-Teacher, a student must be willing to honor Reiki and make it their life's focus, an extreme commitment to Healing and Teaching. She not only taught Reiki, but chose to live it daily as well. It cannot easily be separated.

WHO WAS MASTER TAKATA?

Small Hands Heal Many

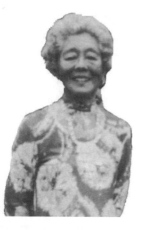

In the Reiki Lineage or heritage known as the "Usui Tradition," there was first the founder, Master Mikao Usui, then Master Chujiro Hayashi, and, in our lineage followed Master Hawayo Kawamura-Takata.

When Master Chujiro Hayashi accepted the charge by Master Usui to preserve and maintain the Reiki Tradition, he had at that time, no knowledge or warning of World War II. In the first Reiki Clinic in Tokyo, Japan, Master Hayashi trained thirteen masters. Before his transition, he initiated Hawayo Takata, a woman, into the mastership and charged her to carry on the Reiki tradition. It seemed knew even before the onset of World War II that Takata would be the only practicing Reiki Master to survive that war, and that she would carry the torch on to America.

It seems ironic that Hayashi's Reiki clinic was the only building in the immediate area to survive the ravages and bombings of the war. After the war, Takata practiced and taught Reiki for forty-five years, moving the center of the Usui System of Natural Healing from Tokyo, Japan to the United States. We owe her much gratitude, not only for saving the Reiki tradition, but also for sharing Reiki with the rest of the world.

Hawayo Kawamuru (Takata) was born December 24, 1900 and made her transition on December 12, 1980. She was the third child born to her parents, cane harvesters, on the island of Kauai, in the newly formed Territory of Hawaii. She was named after this new territory.

At age twelve, Hawayo began working in the cane fields, but the work was so hard and she was so little that she vowed at that time to do something better with her tiny hands. She had no idea at that time that these tiny hands would later hold the great healing power and entire fate of the Usui Reiki Tradition.

Young Hawayo's next job was working as a substitute first grade teacher. She later added to this the responsibility of washing dishes and waiting tables in a soda fountain. She was still herself yet a student then, completing her own studies in a Japanese School. Through her job at the soda fountain, Hawayo met a woman who was a wealthy plantation owner. She offered Hawayo a summer job with her in Kealia. Hawayo remained in her employ for the next twenty-four years. It was while working on the plantation that she met her husband, Saichi Takata, an accountant. They were married March 10, 1917, when Hawayo was sixteen.

Saichi was the first person of Asian descent to be appointed to serve on the district welfare board. They had two daughters, and life seemed good until Saichi began to suffer from ill health. Saichi and Hawayo traveled to the Maeda Clinic in Tokyo where Saichi learned that he had lung cancer. Saichi died in 1930 at the young age of thirty-four. Before his death, he told Hawayo not to grieve for him, that he would always try to be with her, that there is, in truth, no death but merely change, called transition.

Following Saichi's transition, Hawayo worked so hard to keep her family going that she collapsed with a nervous breakdown. She also was suffering from what was later diagnosed as a tumor in the stomach, gallstones and appendicitis. As if this was not bad enough, Hawayo's sister, who was only twenty-five years old, died after four days of contracting tetanus. Although not well, she boarded a steamer bound for Japan. She knew that it was up to her to tell her mother and father, who had returned to their native country, of the sad news of their daughter's death. She carried Saichi's ashes along with her on her journey to Kyoto (former home of Grand Master Usui) for a service at the Ohtani Temple.

After visiting her mother and her father, Hawayo Takata was scheduled for surgery in the Maeda Hospital in Tokyo, where Saichi was treated for his lung cancer. On the way into the operating room, Takata heard a voice urging her again and again to ask the head surgeon if this operation was really necessary. The answer from him was that it would take longer, but perhaps Reiki would prevent the need for surgery. Her faith in that unknown voice led her directly to Hayashi's Reiki Clinic, "Shina No Machi," located just across the street from the Maeda Hospital.

Takata was greeted at the Reiki Clinic by a receptionist who was Dr. Chujiro Hayashi's wife. With her first Reiki Treatment, the warmth flowing from the hands of the two Reiki Practitioners amazed Takata. It was also amazing to her that they were able to diagnose exactly what her physical problems were...tumor, gallstones and appendicitis. Takata, who was raised on an island far away from Japan, had many questions concerning Reiki. She did not understand what Reiki was, or where it came from. Dr. Hayashi told Takata that Reiki came from space like radio waves and was called the Universal Life Force. He further explained to her that it could not be fathomed, and was therefore labeled Reiki. After four days of Reiki treatments, Takata felt worse, but within four months of Reiki treatments, Takata's health was completely restored. She felt compelled to study Reiki in order to keep herself healthy. Many are called to Reiki with the same compelling desire to maintain good health, or to eliminate dis-ease from their lives. It is, after all, not necessary to be ill. Thousands of years ago, a famous Sage from India named Shankara said that "People grow old and die because they see others grow old and die." We embrace the notion of dis-ease because it is a part of our culture, part of what we are raised to believe.

After calling a meeting of the "Usui Light Energy Research Association," Hayashi received permission to teach Reiki to Takata. This was considered unusual because Takata was not only a woman, but also not from Japan, therefore, an outsider. Her payment for learning Reiki was to work as a practitioner in the clinic every day for a year. She was initiated into First Degree Reiki and learned from Master Hayashi to "remove the cause and there shall be no effect." He also taught her about the power of Reiki Consciousness, the evolved state of mind that allowed people to understand that they could be healed without painful surgery if they only allowed themselves to understand and embrace this ancient healing method. At the end of her first year, she was invited to be initiated into Second Degree Reiki. After her initiation, she then returned to Kauai in 1937. It is also speculated that Hayashi initiated both Takata and his wife into the Reiki Mastership before Takata's return to Hawaii. Others say that this initiation took place during Hayashi's visit to Honolulu in 1938. Hayashi did healing and teaching for a short time during his visit there, leaving notice that Takata was to carry on the healing work in the islands that he had started.

It was in 1939 in Hilo, on the big island of Hawaii, that Takata's first healing center was created. On this property she had two rooms for treatment, a waiting room, and living quarters for her family. Her reputation as a healer flourished and she began to travel the islands teaching Reiki as well. This she did until 1940, when a disturbing dream that she had directed her once again to return to Japan to see Master Hayashi. She saw him, in her dream, dressed in a white kimono (robe) preparing for his transition. Her arrival in Japan found Hayashi in good health. He told her that since she was there, she should study hydrotherapy for a few months and then visit before her return to Hawaii.

Master Chujiro Hayashi was increasingly disturbed by his clairvoyant messages of the Great War that he knew was to come. He was also aware that, as a retired naval officer, he would be recalled into active duty in the war. As a Reiki Master and practicing devout Buddhist, he knew that he could not play a part in causing death. He chose, inspite of his good health, to create his transition from the physical plane, in an process of conscious dying. On May 10th, 1941, at the age of sixty-two, dressed in his white silk kimono, Hawashi made his transition, leaving Master Hawayo Kawamura-Takata in charge of preserving and maintaining the Reiki tradition.

Hayashi had informed Takata where to go to be safe from the bombings of Hawaii. She originally had planned to return to take over Hayashi's Clinic after the War, but after visiting the destroyed area where most of the buildings and homes were gone except for the Reiki Clinic, she returned to Hawaii and began to travel and teach throughout most of the United States.

As the demands for more and more Reiki Classes grew, Takata knew that she would have to have help. She was traveling throughout the Hawaiian Islands instructing her hundreds of students there, but demand on the mainland of the United States was growing. After forty years as the only Reiki Master-Teacher, Takata, now in her mid-seventies, decided to initiate others into the responsibility of Master-Teachers of Usui Shiki Ryoho, the Usui School for the Healing Art of Reiki. Before her transition in December of 1980, she initiated twenty-two of her students into the Reiki Mastership as Teachers. The chosen twenty-two masters were the link to Takata, Takata was the link to Hayashi, Hayashi was the link to Usui; Usui brought forth the link to the Universal Life force. See the present need for healing on our dear planet, then see yourself as a vital healing link, connecting to your master and back to Master Usui.

Takata's life on this Earth Plane was not an easy one; she had suffered many hardships, sadness, and physical obstacles. However, she turned these hardships and problems into opportunities for personal and planetary growth. Perhaps the torch of Master Takata burns the brightest in those who have struggled to transform personal tragedies in life into great opportunities for healing through the vital touch of Reiki.

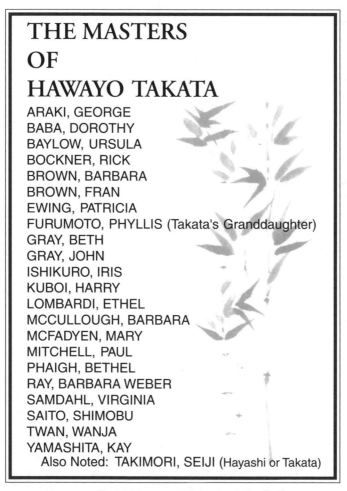

THE MASTERS OF HAWAYO TAKATA

ARAKI, GEORGE
BABA, DOROTHY
BAYLOW, URSULA
BOCKNER, RICK
BROWN, BARBARA
BROWN, FRAN
EWING, PATRICIA
FURUMOTO, PHYLLIS (Takata's Granddaughter)
GRAY, BETH
GRAY, JOHN
ISHIKURO, IRIS
KUBOI, HARRY
LOMBARDI, ETHEL
MCCULLOUGH, BARBARA
MCFADYEN, MARY
MITCHELL, PAUL
PHAIGH, BETHEL
RAY, BARBARA WEBER
SAMDAHL, VIRGINIA
SAITO, SHIMOBU
TWAN, WANJA
YAMASHITA, KAY
   Also Noted: TAKIMORI, SEIJI (Hayashi or Takata)

Toward a New Definition of Healing
for Maintaining Perfect Health

I am very aware that some people are chosen by their tribe to be healers. I am just as aware that there are others who make a conscious decision at some point in their lives to fill a healing role. There is an expansion to this, and that is that I believe that all people have some innate ability to heal, especially to heal themselves. It all has to do with the POWER of the mind, combined with the POWER of the universe. What are you capable of achieving? Positive thinkers believe that you are whatever the mind can conceive of and believe in.

Reiki is a wonderful gift that allows people the connection, as a channel for the Universal Life Force Energy, to finally embrace the notion, to believe that they have become empowered. It gives them permission, without reserve, to be a healing channel. The fact is that many were probably powerful healers in several past life experiences, whether they believe in the possibility of past lives or not.

Reiki also makes people responsible for their own health and well being. They choose to be healthy and focus upon health and fully expect it as a result of their Reiki training. I teach my students of Reiki to live the thought: "I manifest health and prosperity in my life." Reiki empowers people to know that they no longer need to be victims of drifting unawareness, helpless magnets for whatever bug awaits them. They do not have to rely upon Western (allopathic) Medicine to heal dis-ease that has penetrated the physical body, having already passed through the mental, emotional, and spiritual bodies. Edgar Cayce said that treating the physical body without healing the other aspects of the self (the mental, emotional, and spiritual) is like putting a band-aid on a blown tire. The problem will manifest again and again until the consciousness is altered. Thoughts and words have great power and can become a real force in healing. Healing in this expanded sense is being accountable for your own vibrant health. You are directly responsible for your own well-ness, or whatever healing needs to take place. You have the tools with Reiki, and the mind that can keep dis-ease away from you. Healing takes place, if you would, before it is even needed. Healing becomes prevention intervention. In fact, you can choose to eradicate the concept of, and perhaps whatever the need for, dis-ease from your awareness. You may believe that this is not humanly possible. The fact is that there is much more to our abilities than you could ever imagine. We do have the ability to make what we previously may have thought of as impossible, possible. And we can share this gift of healing and these healing thoughts with others. And while we are sharing, let's also share JOY, LOVE, and FORGIVENESS. That is when the real healing begins; when you learn to live in the light of love. The ultimate power is LOVE, the Universal Life Force Energy. That is why Reiki connects to the heart center, why the energy is emerald and the heart center is the same color and vibration. My wish for all who are called to Reiki is that their experience is a joyful one filled with love, light, and peace.

A Torch in Daylight by Reiki Master Karyn K. Mitchell

REI & KI: "SPIRIT TAKING BREATH"
A LOOK BEYOND THE DEFINITION OF
UNIVERSAL LIFE FORCE ENERGY

"Rei" has been defined in Reiki as Universal Life Force. That is what I was taught in Reiki Level One. While I do not reject this part of the definition, I would like to add that I believe that the word "Universal" lacks soul or spirit, since the divinity has been either disqualified or omitted in the Western translation process. The Japanese character for "Rei" is more intrinsically defined as spirit, soul, divine, sacred or even miraculous.

Then what does Ki mean? Ki is an important part of oriental culture, including medicine, art, philosophy, and physical training. Only by experiencing Ki, can a person begin to understand it, as the full significance of Ki is clarified only through personal experience. The problem in even writing about Ki, is that there is no English equivalent, no adequate words or phrases that translate well from "Ki" into English. In a sense, to condense Ki to a simple definition or words, places limitation on what it actually is. According to the ancient Taoists, Ki is the crucial indicator of life. Without Ki life does not exist. Is Ki then the connection that we might call Spirit? Or, in this same sense, then, is Ki more closely associated with the Hindu term "Prana," which means life energy, or life principle of the Universe? Prana, it is believed, is a nutritive subtle energy that is taken in during the process of breathing. This subtle energy is energy that exists separate or outside of ordinary time and space, much like electromagnetic energy moves faster than the speed of light. This subtle energy moves through the human meridian system once taken in by the body.

The Subtle Universal Law And The Integral Way Of Life, by Taoist Master NI HUA CHING, he describes Chi (or Ki) in the following Manner:

"Chi is the vital universal energy which composes, permeates and moves through everything that exists. Chi may be defined as the ultimate cause, and, at the same time, the ultimate effect. When chi conglomerates, it is called matter. When chi is diffuse, it is called space. When chi animates form, it is called life. When chi separates and withdraws from form it is called death. When chi flows, there is health. When chi is blocked, there is sickness and disease. Chi embraces all things, circulates through and sustains them. The Nei-ching says, 'In heaven there is chi and on earth form. When the two interplay there is life.'"

It is difficult to define life, so we must learn to be expansive, and think beyond what we have always known and been able to explain.

The Chinese call this Ki, Qi or Chi, and perceive of it functionally, in five different ways, by what it does in conjunction with the body's ability to move:

1.) It includes physical and mental movement, like running, thinking, and even growing up.
2.) It acts as an immune system, protecting the body.
3.) It changes food into blood.
4.) It holds in place vital organs and keeps the blood in its proper path way. (Blood flows through blood vessels and meridians; there is not much distinction between the two.)
5.) It maintains warmth in the body. These various types of Qi, Ki, or Chi, are subject to what the Chinese call Yin or Yang "disharmonies," (stagnant, deficient or excess Qi), what we would call lack of balance or perhaps even, dis-ease.

This brings us to a greater understanding of the way that Master Mikao Usui performed Reiki in the streets of Japan. As I have mentioned, he carried a torch in daylight to "raise the consciousness" or vibration of the "shen" or spirit. He would then observe, "take a pulse" and heal. The pulse is taken at acupuncture points (on major meridians), but the primary one, and probably the one that Master Usui utilized, was the prominent point at the radial artery near the wrist. Pulse taken can define primary disharmonies that may exist in the body. There are various types of pulses: floating pulse and sinking pulse (depth of pulse), full pulse and empty pulse (strength of pulse), rapid pulse and slow pulse (speed of pulse), big (broad) pulse and thin pulse (width of pulse), slippery and choppy pulse as well as wiry and light pulse (shape of pulse), short pulse and long pulse (length of pulse), knotted, hurried and intermittent pulse (rhythm of pulse), and there are other aspects of measuring pulse such as: moderate pulse, flooding pulse, minute pulse, frail pulse, soggy pulse, leather pulse, hidden pulse, confined pulse, spinning bean pulse, scattered pulse, and hollow pulse. These patterns were used to help diagnose what needed healed in the body.

While the pulse was Master Usui's way of discerning what needed attention in the body, the meridian system was also the pathway for healing energies to follow. Master Usui's healing method was in a non-clinical environment. (It was, after all, Master Hayashi who brought Reiki in from the streets and into a purely clinical setting; he also set the hand placements much like we use today: four on the head, four on the front of the body and four on the back.) When we work with the chakra system, are we working with a completely different system than the meridian or pulse system originally utilized by Master Usui? Both are energy channels; in the chakras, energy flows in through a system of petals called nadis. In the center of each chakra is a stem that connects it to a most important energy channel called "Sushumna," that follows the spine from the base to the top of the head. The "Ida" (lunar or cool energy) and "Pingala" (solar or heat energy carrier) are also energy channels. Pingala begins on the right side of the root chakra and ends in the upper right nostril; the Ida begins on the left of the root chakra and ends in the left nostril. These channels, the Sushumna, the Ida, and the Pingala act as senders and receivers of subtle energies, and must be open and work harmoniously for a sense of well being. The three separate channels meet or intersect at six different locations along the spinal column, each forming the six main or axis chakras. There is one more connection, at the brain. This is the crown chakra. Since the chakras are meridian intersections, we are essentially using the same system, working with the chakras, and through them, accessing the merdian system.

It is interesting to note that as a person's vibrational rate increases, with what we call spiritual development, the chakras extend out further than the normal four inches in all directions. As these chakras extend out further, the frequency of the vibrations also increase. It is in this manner that what we could consider a spiritually advanced person can harmoniously effect the environment by sharing Light energies.

I would like to share, then, a few simple re-definitions of Reiki for you to reflect upon: SPIRIT LIGHT, SOUL ILLUMINATION, SCARED LIGHT (or LIFE) FORCE, or even perhaps DIVINE BREATH or SPIRIT TAKING BREATH. The term, KIMUSUBJI, means when the Ki" of a man and the Ki of a woman unite, a new being or life can be created.

The term Universal Life Force, as the Western definitions of Reiki, comes from a desire to take the Spirit or Divine Nature out of Reiki, and this is not possible. While Reiki is not a religion, this does not imply that we negate our connection to ALL THAT IS, regardless of what you call the ALL. It is, after all, what we channel, and it is Spiritual, a Sacred Light, a light for raising consciousness (illumination) for healing, much like Master Usui's torch in daylight.

My experience with Reiki is a spiritual connection to ALL THAT IS, it is Spirit Taking Breath, or physical form connection to ALL THAT IS through the force of the Spirit. Without spirit what are we? And without Spirit, what is Reiki? Traditional Reiki is spiritual Reiki.

A final consideration of the definition of Reiki is born of the martial arts tradition. "Rei" means respect. "Ki" is all life in its many forms. The definition when integrated means "respect for all life," not just human life, but all living things.

THE TIBETAN LAMAS

Reiki as a system of healing was re-discovered by Master Usui in the late 1800's. The word "Reiki," is a Japanese term that Master Usui created in an attempt to label the healing energy system, the connecting link, or anchor, of energy from All That Is (or the Tao) to the physical realm of humanity.

It is important to note that this 2,500 (plus) year old system was not always called "Reiki." This label, again, came with the re-discovery of the attunement process by Master Usui on sacred Mount Kuri Yama, where he meditated and fasted for twenty-one days until he was presented with the four symbols or calligraphs that are utilized in the physical Usui Shiki Ryoho sysem. Master Usui was charged to preserve and protect the sacred knowledge and wisdom revealed to him, and then pass this on to another in the physical to preserve and protect its future.

The anchoring of the healing energies to the physical, called implanting, is shrouded in mystery, as is much that surpasses the physical/mental capacities of human understanding. It is much like any knowledge of our past, or history, if you would. There is the written, mental account of what happened in the past, but that is not all that happened. There is a history that transcends the written word, a history above or beyond history, a history that is apparent only to those whose consciousness is expanded enough to comprehend the Truth. So the true origin of the connection to the Universal Life Force or All That Is, or what Master Usui called "Reiki" comes from the same source as humanity. Some accounts about Reiki speculate that this original source is Pleiadian, some say it is Enochian, from the Angelic realms of St. Michael, or from the priestly order of Melchizedek, and I have also heard that it was Atlantean, but lost to us during the deconstructing of the DNA. The source is what we would call Divinely Inspired, or beyond ourselves in Third Dimension Reality. It is the desire of the individual to transcend the self to bring about peace, balance, and healing on all levels, and then to share this discovery with others. The historical beginnings that we can account for begin with the Tibetan Holy Lamas. When it was time for the Initiate to integrate the heart and mind as one, this readied Initiate was led to a sacred place, a temple or cave, where they were instructed to sit and contemplate inscriptions written in copper on a wall in front of them. As they meditated, these sacred geometric designs or mandalas would vibrate at a frequency that had a molecular-magnetic influence upon the neurokinetic system of the body.

After days or weeks of meditation and fasting, the Initiate would become one with the sacred symbols; the symbols would then be implanted in the consciousness. A master became the physical embodiment of the sacred symbols as living energies. Some Initiates were more receptive than others, some received the attunement faster and with a stronger influence.

The same is true today as well. There must exist the consciousness for readiness; many are called to the sacred spiritual path of Reiki, those who are open to the energies gain great understanding and expanded awareness. These are the ones who understand that what is essential to life is invisible to the eye. The physical is exhaustible, the spiritual is eternal. If your definition of life is purely tied to the physical, there you will remain, grounded to the Earth Plane. If you connect to the Spiritual then you can truly be free and transcend pain and fear.

THE MERIDIAN SYSTEM AND KI

Ki flows through the body through the Meridian System. Meridians are invisible channels, not the blood vessels themselves. These meridians connect the inner body with the outer body. A disharmony along a meridian may manifest in the organ corresponding to that meridian. This chart shows the approximate time that the meridians flow. If you notice any discomfort consistently during the day or awakening during the night, it may be due to the flow of that particular meridian. The flow of Ki is not in harmony, and it is affecting the organ corresponding to that meridian.

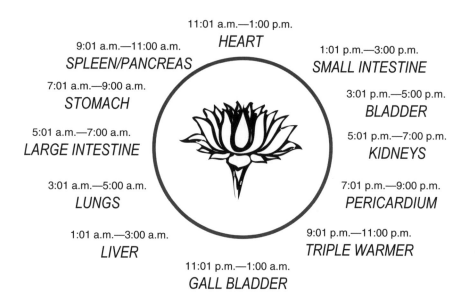

11:01 a.m.—1:00 p.m.
HEART

9:01 a.m.—11:00 a.m.
SPLEEN/PANCREAS

1:01 p.m.—3:00 p.m.
SMALL INTESTINE

7:01 a.m.—9:00 a.m.
STOMACH

3:01 p.m.—5:00 p.m.
BLADDER

5:01 a.m.—7:00 a.m.
LARGE INTESTINE

5:01 p.m.—7:00 p.m.
KIDNEYS

3:01 a.m.—5:00 a.m.
LUNGS

7:01 p.m.—9:00 p.m.
PERICARDIUM

1:01 a.m.—3:00 a.m.
LIVER

9:01 p.m.—11:00 p.m.
TRIPLE WARMER

11:01 p.m.—1:00 a.m.
GALL BLADDER

A Torch in Daylight by Reiki Master Karyn K. Mitchell

WHAT IS THE ATTUNEMENT/INITIATION PROCESS IN REIKI?

According to The American Heritage Dictionary of the English Language, to attune means to bring into harmony. Initiation means "a ceremony, ritual, or period of instruction with which a new member is admitted to an organization, office, or knowledge." To help a student understand the purpose or intention of the attunement/initiation process in Reiki, we must first guide them to understand their reasons for taking Reiki in the first place. It is a commitment that must be considered from the standpoint of personal growth on the spiritual, mental, emotional, and physical levels.

When a person has fear about the attunement/initiation process itself, I ask that they meditate concerning the source of that fear. Perhaps it is a fear that they are about to engage in some type of subversive or counter-religious (or religious) act. Those of us who have been through the attunements know that this is absolutely not the case. Overcoming fear, if fear is there, helps the student to gain personal power. But overcoming fear is not the real purpose of the attunement process. The attunement process is to raise the vibration of the individual and connect them to the source of limitlessness. The more open the individual is to the attunement, the higher the vibration that will be allowed to flow to them. In other words, the degree that they can embrace the potential of the attunement is the degree of power that they will allow and create space for in their lives. That is why it is important that all students coming to Reiki understand what Reiki is and does. Knowledge melts fear.

The attunement ceremony is uplifting and spiritual in the sense that it affirms a belief in the power of the self. It does bring harmony and peace through a greater understanding of healing. Reiki is one of the few, if not the only, healing modality where self-healing is possible. Healing knowledge is an inherent part of the new member instruction that comes with the attunement. So if the attunement process discourages a student from taking Reiki, then perhaps that student was not quite ready yet to make the commitment or changes that Reiki brings. We must honor the path of the hesitant as well as that of the enthusiastic.

During the First Degree Reiki Class, I do a guided meditation prior to the attunement/initiation. One of the elements that I bring into this meditation is an acceptance of a gift from the Masters. The gift comes in a beautiful gold or silver box that must be opened. The wonderful gift, once accepted by the initiate, is of course, a symbol of Reiki itself. It is also love.

Reiki 1 ATTUNEMENT PROCEDURE

meditation:

Prior to the Reiki I initiation, you will be guided in a meditation that prepares you spiritually to become a channel for the Reiki energies. During the course of this meditation, you may have the opportunity to meet your personal spiritual guides.

Your Physical, Mental, Emotional and Spiritual bodies are etherically cleansed during the meditation.

We may also begin to work with your chakras ...starting with the 1st (Root), 2nd (Sacral), 3rd (Solar Plexus), 4th (Heart Chakra ... but not the heart itself), 5th (Throat), 6th (Pineal, Third Eye, or Eye of Shiva), and the 7th (Crown).

initiation process:

It is important to remove all jewelry, watches, and barrettes prior to all attunements.

Your chairs are placed in a circle with the backs toward the middle. This is to create a mirror effect and will facilitate in creating a greater connection to the energies.

You will close your eyes and put yourself in a meditative state. I will place my hands on your shoulders to connect with your energies. Then I will place energies above your Crown, and tap you on the shoulder. I ask that you lift your hands in Namaste, prayer or palms touching position, above and in front of your forehead. I will blow across your Crown and then clap the outside of your hands. Then I will lift and align your chakras.

Next I present energy to the Third Eye. I ask that when I tap your shoulder, you place your hands, again in palms touching position, in front of the Third Eye where I will blow into your Third Eye area and then clap the outside of your hands. This is repeated for the Throat and the Heart Centers. Then I will go behind you and lift and align your chakras once again.

Please remain in a meditative state until all have shared the initiation process. When the bell rings, you may open your eyes and join hands in a circle facing the center.

You have now been empowered with the gift of Reiki 1.

Please note: Attunement procedures differ among Masters and lineages.

The energy transfer opens you up to the universal Reiki energy. This also initiates the 21 day clearing cycle of the seven major chakras, one chakra a day, starting at the Root, processing through each three times. The initiation and clearing cycle opens you to healing and psychic channels. You become more balanced after the completion of the process. (See Clearing Process, page 28.)

white light, clearing negativity:

Once you become one with Reiki, you are one with the light. The light is within you and around you. Reiki is love, and it can never be used for anything but divine good. However, until you fully realize this, you may desire to further surround yourself with other protective light such as blue or white light. You can visualize this as a switch in your Solar Plexus area that you can turn on to protect yourself from all negativity. This is true for all types of negative energies. We also sweep the auric field of the client, front and back, whisking the negativity into the etheric garbage can for transmutation.

chakra spinning:

In the second part of the Reiki I class, you will be taught the hand placements and also be taught how to align and spin the chakras. This can be done with a crystal or pendulum on a chain of at least six inches. Starting at the Crown Chakra, we will check the vortex of each chakra and bring it into further balance during the Reiki class treatment. You will be guided to learn how to do this procedure for others.

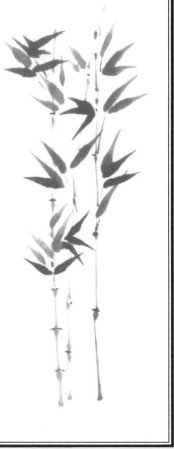

THE TWENTY-ONE DAY CLEARING PROCESS
Honor the Opportunity for Soul Growth

I like to compare the initiation process in Reiki to a vortex of Universal Energy pouring into the Crown Chakra. At each level of attunement, the vibratory rate is heightened, and you are able to tap into a higher, wider channel of that Universal Energy. Some may experience this shift immediately, expanded color consciousness, a buzzing or heightened sensitivity in the crown center, or a sense of floating or light headedness. (It is important to remember to remove all jewelry, watches, and barrettes prior to any attunement as metals may create disharmony in the chakra areas.)

In order for the vibratory rate to be raised with each attunement, there has to be a clearing of old patterns and thoughts that inhibit the growth of the consciousness. This clearing takes place in an orderly fashion, proceeding up the axis chakras one by one: week one consists of one day each for the chakra center of the Root, Sacral, Solar Plexus, Heart, Throat, Third Eye, and then the Crown. Week two begins at the Root Chakra and proceeds day by day up to the Crown Center. Week three is a repeat of the other two. This is the same cycle and procedure for healing acute dis-ease in others. It is best if they are treated for twenty-one days straight to clear the chakras three times each in order to remove old patterns and pain. I like to compare this chakra healing (clearing) process to a check mark. You have to go down before you can go up. This process may prove to be uncomfortable for many people. As the blocks that are preventing your progress are brought forward, they are released by your Physical, Emotional, Mental, and Spiritual bodies. The effects that you may experience are widespread, and could range from irritability and crying to the inability to eat low

. You may also be unable to toler- Please keep in mind that this pro-. What you may feel as various ng the twenty-one day clearing or ore space for transcendence. You an's Death, so to speak, to go far nement is life-altering. Many Stu- Level One Reiki clears issues con- o clears issues of relationships with clears issues with relationships with nd all life.

ce the twenty-one day clearing cycle y for soul growth. Honor the process and be kind to you. Do self-treatment every day, and be sure to drink six to eight glasses of pure water daily. This does not include tea, coffee, or any other water-based beverage. You may wish to refer to some of the suggestions on the next page. It may also be useful to repeat the Reiki Principles to yourself, "Just for today do not anger. Just for today do not worry. Honor your parents, teachers, and elders. Earn your living honestly. Show gratitude to every living thing." Living "just for today," you focus on the NOW. Anger and fear are replaced by love as your vibratory rate and consciousness are raised. But the shift is not always without pain or letting go of old patterns; in Reiki we call this releasing of old patterns, the Twenty-one Day Clearing Process. You will be lifted even higher when the transformation is complete. You may not recognize the new you at first, but trust me, you will never want to go back to that old self again.

Reiki YOUR MIND AND BODY

◆   **M**editate for 10-15 minutes three times a day. <u>CLEAR YOUR MIND COM-PLETELY</u> ahead of time. Tell your mental/physical bodies that they will have time later to chatter...not during meditation. MEDITATION is essential to re-store balance and to ALLOW yourself time to just BE.

◆   **G**o to bed before 11:00 PM, but do not sleep too much, as this stagnates energy in the body. <u>Exercise</u> and fresh air also helps.

◆   **D**rink eight or more glasses of pure water a day, at least. Herb teas...(Echinacea is my favorite to stimulate the immune system) are also a great help, but drink without sweetener and avoid aluminum spoons and utensils.

◆   **A**void at all costs florescent lights, crowds and loud noises. Classical or free flowing music is helpful and relaxing.

◆   **A**void negative thoughts and negative people. If you are forced to listen to any type of negativity, cross your legs and cross your fingers so that it will not penetrate your aura. Also try to avoid the media news reports on television, radio, and in the newspaper. You're especially vulnerable at this time to mood swings, so try to keep things positive and upbeat.

◆   **I**f you feel drained of energy, you need to look around at your environment for any negativity. Do some mental housekeeping...sweep out any thoughts, nega-tive people, or old patterns of behavior that drag you down. They no longer serve you. Look at what you do every moment during the day. Does everything you do reflect and honor who you are now spiritually? Listen to that still small voice inside of you. It may direct you to any energy leaks.

◆   **A** quick boost for lack of energy is to imagine that you have an energy switch in your solar plexus, just above the navel. If you are in need of a quick burst of energy, flip that switch upward and imagine a flash of brilliant white and electric blue pulsing through your physical body, renewing and restoring your energy. Hold your hand on or above the navel. Do not use this more that a couple of times a day, however. This is also good to protect your aura from outside nega-tive influences.

◆   **H**onor yourself. Think loving thoughts towards yourself, and even do as Louise Hay suggests look in the mirror and affirm your beauty as a person and your love for yourself often. We have the power. We cannot wait for, or expect others to affirm our beauty, strength, and love.

◆   **K**now that you have an important purpose. You have been called to Reiki for a reason. You have a vital and necessary role to help restore the planet. You are clearing old negativity to make way for the new you, a you that you and others will love and respect more than you ever imagined. Thank the process for its healing and growth.

◆   **R**ead. Study. Take your mind to places it's never been before!

What is a Healing Crisis?

A "Healing Crisis" is a positive sign in the physical body, but it can create fear in a client who does not know that such a crisis is different than a dis-ease crisis.

Reiki speeds up the healing processes. An acute dis-ease that would take two to three weeks to run its course in the body, for example, would be accelerated with a Reiki Treatment. This same dis-ease might take four days to a week, but in accelerating the healing process, the client may feel suddenly worse. You should reassure your client that this is not only natural, but constructive. Every organ in the body is eliminating waste products to pave the way for cellular regeneration. Since this is the case, there may be fever or cold/flu-like symptoms. All other elimination in the body remains regular, thereby cleansing and purifying the system.

In a dis-ease crisis, the opposite is true, and constipation or diarrhea may be a result of systemic malfunction. The blood stream carries toxins thrown off by one organ to another; the same blood that feeds and bathes the spleen also feeds and bathes the heart. Approximately 125 barrels of blood go throughout the entire organism.

There can be a mental healing crisis as well as a physical one. In such cases, there may be severe reflection upon the past, which creates fear, anger, or depression. There have been reports of clients who related incidents that occurred twenty or thirty years prior. Such psychic clearing is perhaps more valuable than the physical healing; what it does is to eliminate the root cause of a probable dis-ease in progress. Congested emotions should be treated as open wounds. As practitioners of healing, we can provide comfort in such emotional crisis, and again, assure our client that recognizing such emotional pain is natural. They should embrace the opportunity to allow these feelings to clear, the tears of sadness actually contain different chemicals than the tears of happiness, yet both are valuable for a balanced life.

In Natural Healing, we embrace the Healing Crisis as self-adjustment. We do not suppress the process with Reiki, we enhance it. If we are working within the Natural Healing System, then we will potentially create a Healing Crisis.

There is another phenomenon that occurs with natural healing. This is what is called retracing. As we reverse the processes of dis-ease, we may continue back, or retrace past dis-eases as well. All of the symptoms of these may be exhibited in the healing crisis. Again, this process which brings back the troubles of the past, should be embraced as part of the healing (clearing) process. It is the time for these to be healed and no longer suppressed in the system.

According to "Hering's Law of Cure," symptoms should disappear from above downward; from within to outward; and in the reverse order of their coming. When this is complete, the client should be free of dis-ease and its symptoms, and in a much better state of health.

REIKI HAND POSITIONS

As a beginning Reiki practitioner, you may desire to have specific guidance concerning the placement of hands during a Reiki treatment. I always tell my students, however, that it is important that they begin to listen to and follow their own intuition in this matter. Takata, for example, taught each student to begin in a different place, but emphasized that it was important to pay special attention to what she called the big motor, the solar plexus/sacral area.

I like to make my energy connection with the client at the head; there I can tell how much stress that the person has brought with them. If there is much stress involved, I ask the client to take three long, slow, deep breaths and as they exhale, release all of the tension, cares, and concerns of the day ... just let go. I place a tissue over the eyes if they like, and gently smooth it over the forehead as if erasing tension. Get yourself into a meditative state of mind and always be sure to remove all of your own personal jewelry, especially watches, as well as any that the client may be wearing that might obstruct the flow of energy. Be certain that neither the client nor you have legs or arms crossed; for your own comfort, maintain good posture and soft knees.

Always try to maintain physical contact with the client so that they know exactly where you are. Adjust your pressure so that it is light and pleasant at all times ... especially at the joint areas or on the face. Be sure to wash hands before beginning and between each client. <u>Also remember to close your fingers (Reiki off)</u> after each treatment is complete. Reiki Masters in particular should clear the minds and keep their eyes open and focused on the client, as the eyes have healing power.

Fingers together at all times, you may begin one of two places: at the crown or at the forehead.

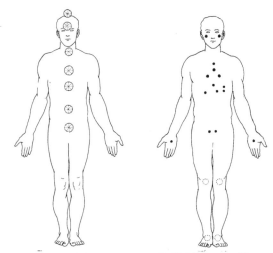

　A Torch in Daylight by ℞eíkí Master Karyn K. Mitchell

Reiki hand positions

body front

1. HEAD
- forehead
- across the eyes/sinuses, be mindful of the nose
- sides of cheek/ears
- cup hands away from throat

2. HEART CHAKRA
- Men: hands side by side
- Women: hands front & back

3. ARMS/HANDS
- lifting arm, place your same forearm beneath theirs, your palm under theirs
- place your other arm gently on theirs

4. BODY TRUNK
- below chest: hands side by side or front to back
- abdomen, same as chest
- hands toward root chakra
- one hand each side of hips

5. LEGS
- one hand each thigh or both hands on each side
- knees, one hand on each knee cap or cup both around one

6. ANKLES
- same as knee joint

7. FEET
- cup or cover, or place hands on both feet bottoms

8. SWEEP AURA
- three times, head to foot

body back

1. BACK OF HEAD

2. NECK

3. SHOULDERS

4. BETWEEN SHOULDERS

5. ONE HAND EACH SIDE OF SPINE DESCEND TO BASE: (Optional: Return and go down spine)

6. THIGH one hand on each

7. KNEE BACK (if not cupped in front)

8. CALF (one hand on each)

9. BACKS OF ANKLES

10. FEET BOTTOM (if neglected in front)

11. SWEEP AURA (three times head to foot)

12. One hand on neck base, other hand on spine base, then walk hands up spine base to neck

13. Pull down walking fingers each side of spine or (optional: squiggle fingers down each side of spine)

Please note: Hand positions may vary with Master and lineage.

Reiki HAND PLACEMENT for TABLE TREATMENT

START BODY FRONT

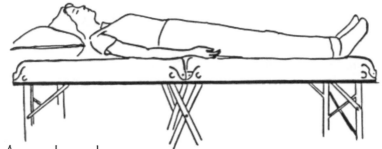

1st Area head

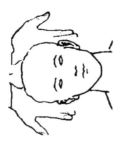

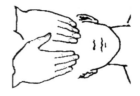

1. palms on crown and fingers wrap toward ears

2. across eyes & sinuses.

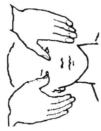

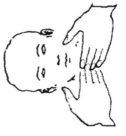

3. cup around temples

4. hands cup above throat.

A Torch in Daylight by Reiki Master Karyn K. Mitchell

2nd Area upper chest & arms

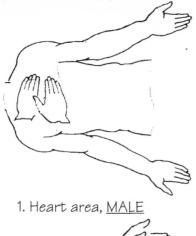

1. Heart area, <u>MALE</u>

2. Heart area, <u>FEMALE</u>

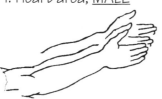

NOTE: Limbs are not treated in some traditions of Reiki.

3. arms, one at a time sandwich their arm in between yours

3rd Area trunk, abdomen, solar plexus and hips

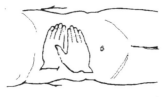

1. trunk upper lower chest

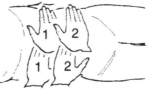

2. trunk lower above navel, abdomen below navel

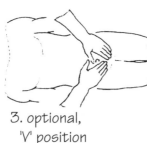

3. optional, 'V' position

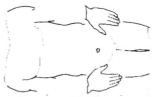

4. on side of upper thighs, (or from back)

4th Area legs, knees, ankles and feet

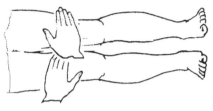

1. thighs hand position 1

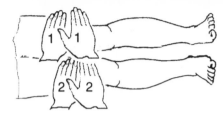

1a. thighs hand position 2

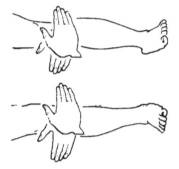

2. Knees, cup hands
   around then do
   ankles and feet

SWEEPING the AURA

Do this three times sweeping from head
 to feet, hands perpendicular to body.

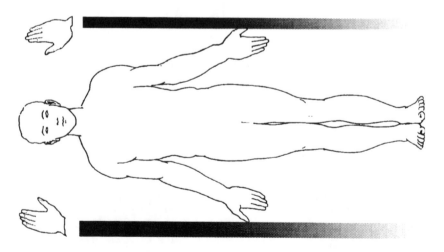

Reiki HAND PLACEMENTS

BODY BACK

1st Area back of head & neck

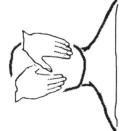 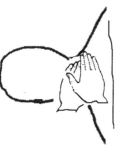

1. palms down on
back of head.

2. palms down on
back of neck.

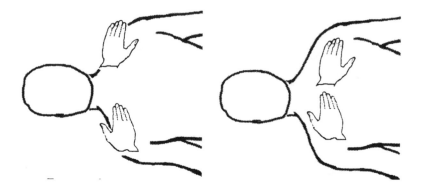

3. top of shoulders
cup around.

3a. or top of shoulders

2nd Area spine

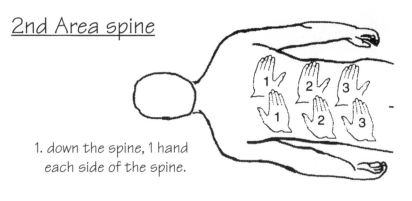

1. down the spine, 1 hand
   each side of the spine.

3rd Area thighs & knees

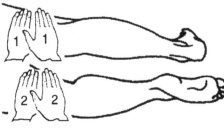
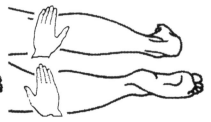

1. palms down on back of thigh.   2. palms down on back of knees.

4th Area calf, ankles & Feet

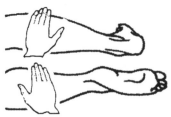
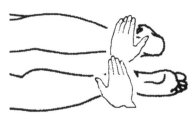

1. palms down on calf.   2. palms cupped around ankles

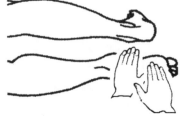

3. palms down on <u>BOTTOM</u> of feet.

A Torch in Daylight by **R**e**í**k**í M**aster **K**aryn **K. M**itchell

Reiki HAND PLACEMENTS for TREATMENTS

SWEEPING THE AURA

Do this three times sweeping from head to feet.

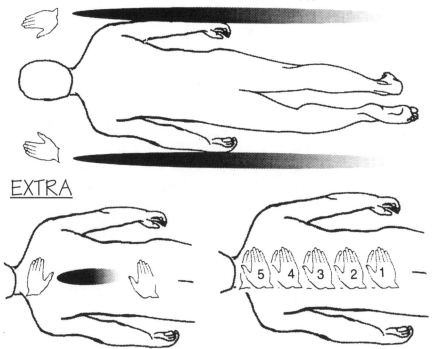

EXTRA

1. palms down, left hand at top 7th cervical vertebrae of back and right hand on sacrum at bottom of back then sense the "fluorescent tube" of light.

Note: Illustrations are for standing on left side of client's body.

1a. walk up the spine, start with both hands flat and thumbs touching, tip right hand up (little finger down, thumb up) bring or slide hand to left thumb, tip left hand (little finger down, thumb up) lower right thumb to left little finger slide left to flat continue procedure all the way up the spine.
Lightly touch head three times, polish halo three times, and pull down bladder meridian, three times with Index and third finger.

Reiki Hand Placements

for Body Front Table Treatment Part I

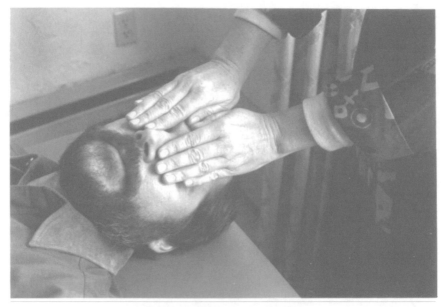

1. Forehead, Eyes

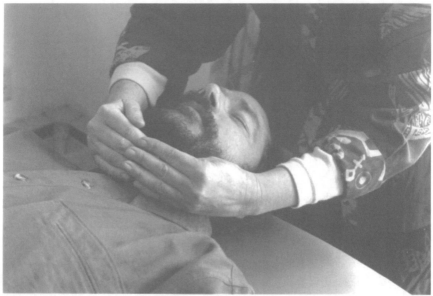

2. Throat Center

A Torch in Daylight by **Reiki Master Karyn K. Mitchell**

Reiki Hand Placements
for Body Front Table Treatment Part II

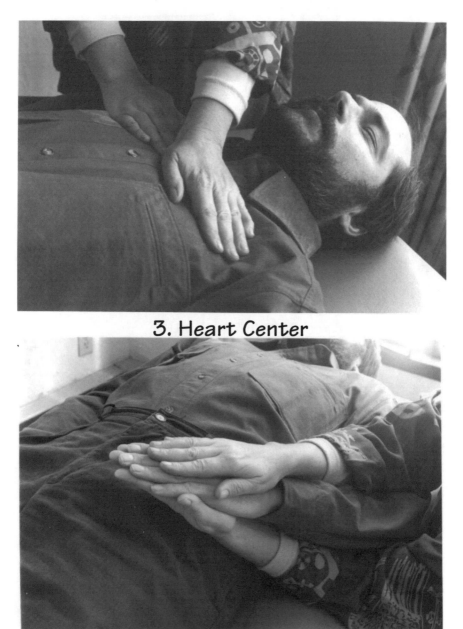

3. Heart Center

4. Hand-Arm Cradle (each side)

Reiki Hand Placements
for Body Front Table Treatment Part III

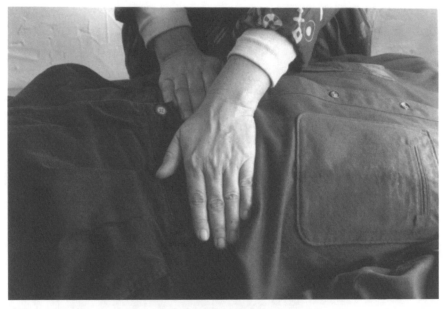

5. Solar Plexus

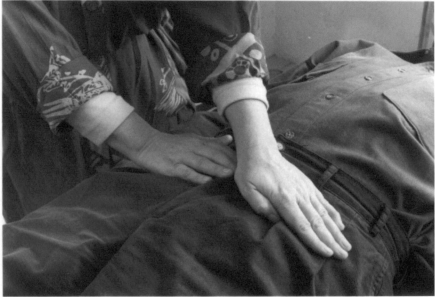

6. Sacral Center

A Torch in Daylight by Reiki Master Karyn K. Mitchell

Reiki Hand Placements
for Body Front Table Treatment Part IV

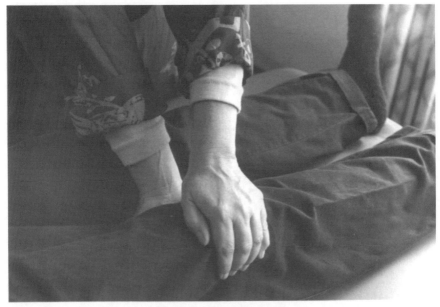

7. Knee Cradle

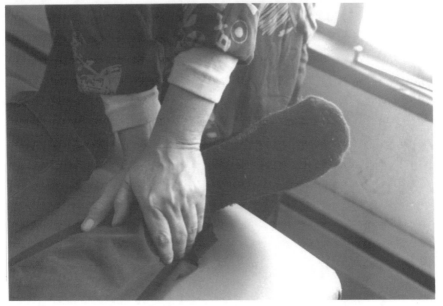

8. Ankle Front

Reiki Hand Placements

for Body Back Table Treatment Part V

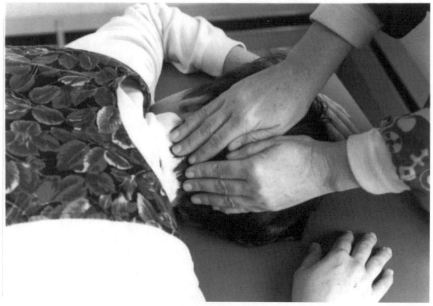

9. Head

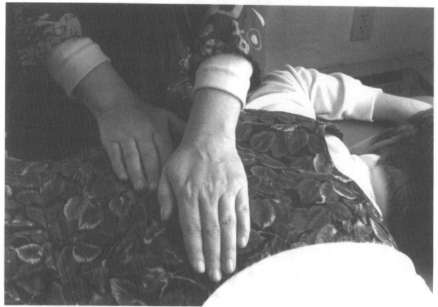

10. Shoulders...then Upper Back

A Torch in Daylight by Reiki Master Karyn K. Mitchell

Reiki Hand Placements
for Body Back Table Treatment Part VI

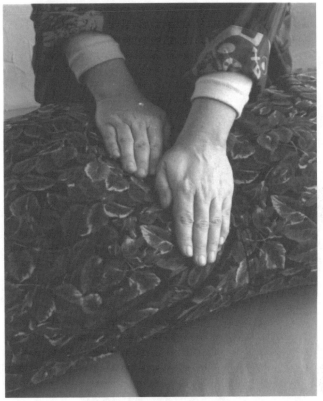

11. Lower Back

REMEMBER:
YOUR WORDS HAVE POWER!

When working with a client during a table treatment, always use a gentle touch, maintaining body contact at all times. Observe Noble Silence!

If your client asks questions, remember to use positive words that promote only love and good health. Your words have power, so use that power to heal. Consider your words carefully if you must speak.

Reiki Hand Placements
for Body Back Table Treatment Part VII

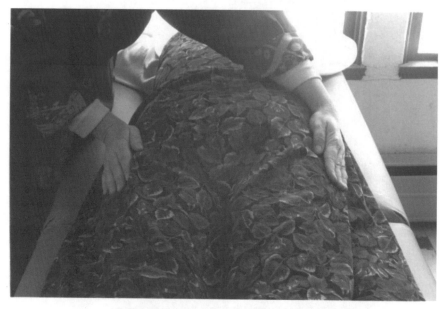

12. Root Center (sides)

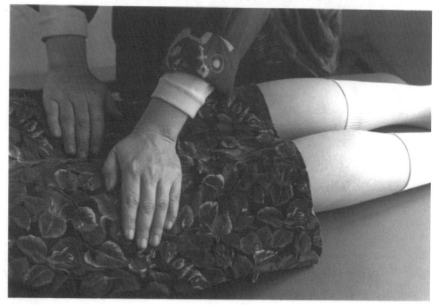

13. Thighs

A Torch in Daylight by Reiki Master Karyn K. Mitchell

Reiki Hand Placements

for Body Back Table Treatment Part VIII

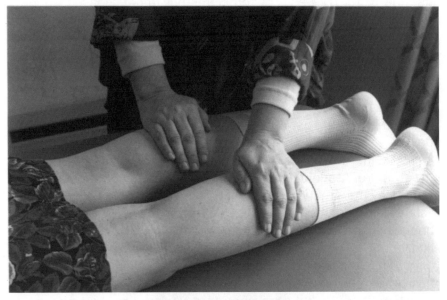

14. Calf of Legs

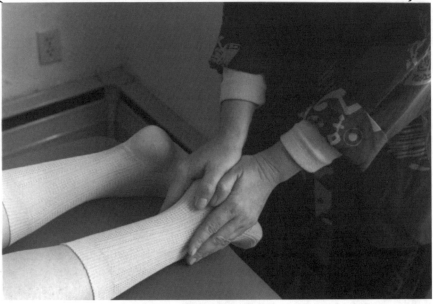

15. Foot

Words To Avoid

As Reiki Practitioners, it is most advantageous to use only positive words when we address a client. In other words, I choose not to use the word "dis-ease" or "problem," but rather "healing opportunity" or "focus." I also try not to use the words "pain" or hurt," as that seems to draw energy and attention to the healing opportunity. We must transcend or move beyond the Western, allopathic model, and focus energy and attention to what is right about the person, rather than what is wrong. That gentle, subtle shift is what reframes the way that a person may be thinking of themselves. Instead of thinking of themselves as wounded, they can focus upon wellness of being.

Other words that we must avoid are "diagnose," "prescribe," "treat," "cure," "patient," and any organ name. These words are copyrighted by the American Medical Association, and do not fit in a holistic healer's paradigm anyway. Chester P. Yozwick states in his booklet, "Legal and Administrative Aspects of a Holistic Health Practice:"

"Watching your language is the most important aspect of this profession. Someone may call you on the phone to ask you questions about what type of service you render. You may never know who is on the other end of the line, so please be mindful not to use any A.M.A. copyrighted words...in place of diagnose, you should get into the habit of using the word evaluate or analyze. In place of the word "treat," use the words that apply. In place of the word cure, use heal. In place of disease, use (problem or affliction*)."

*Again I suggest the words "focus" or "healing opportunity."

Dr. Yozwick states that "No law exists which can prohibit you from maintaining a position of consultant/counselor. Regardless of which state you live in, these licensing laws do not affect you if you work as a consultant. In fact, no license is usually required for holistic health counselors because the area of practice is NOT regulated." (p.32) However, since so much attention is now upon holistic health practitioners, I suggest that you simply be aware of city, county, or state ordinances that may have been enacted since this was written.

I have always felt that if the United States or any governing body herein makes it illegal for consenting adults to touch each other, we are no longer free individuals. I do know that many Professional Reiki Practitioners become ministers of healing churches in order to circumvent controversy. (See information about classes page 152.)

Physical, Emotional, Mental & Spiritual

Physical Body

How do you use your physical body—exercise, awareness, touch? What is the importance of water and outdoor elements of earth to you?

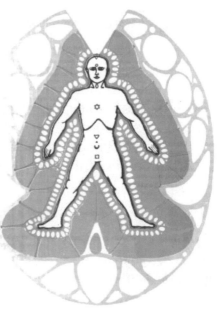

Emotional Body

How do you use your emotional energy? According to Tibetan medicine, there are over 38,000 affective emotions that can cause disease. What fears are you working through——fear of death, fear of being left out, rejection, fear of loss, or change. How can you open to more joy in your life and learn to express your positive emotions?

Mental Body

Are you able to use your mind to further your spiritual goals, or is your mind constantly in the way of you getting things done. Look at how you use your mind and how you can use it for peace and spiritual evolution.

Spiritual Body

How important is your spiritual life? Are you focused on it? Begin to look at your soul's journey into the light and at the path of your spiritual evolution. You evolve more spiritually through meditation and compassion.

ReIKI CHAKRAS

FIRST CHAKRA -ROOT - RED

The first chakra is associated with the body, which includes all the physical senses. Look at anything that comes up around the area of soul's purpose and how you are living in the present moment. Learn to initiate and not just react, don't take simple situations as life-threatening, develop and try new things, become more sensitive to other people's feelings and to not feel separate or different from other people.

SECOND CHAKRA - SACRAL - ORANGE

This chakra concerns how you create and manifest in life. Create original ideas. What you desire for your life is initiated and later actualized.

THIRD CHAKRA - SOLAR PLEXUS - YELLOW

This chakra is the ego and power center, it is concerned with making your life happen. How do you use your ego and power? How can you open to being more powerful and effective? Learn to be your own authority, learn to use power effectively, and learn to link the soul-self with the ego.

FOURTH CHAKRA - HEART - GREEN

This chakra relates to love, safety in the world, faith and self-belief. It deals with attachment and detachment, the need to feel secure, validated, and loved. Learn to go inward for that sense of wholeness instead of turning to others. Look at the energy of love in your heart. Are you secure? How is your level of self-esteem and can you be open to more love in your life? Do you love self and others unconditionally?

FIFTH CHAKRA - THROAT - BLUE

This is the mind and Throat Chakra - concerned with expression of self through the voice and the mind. It deals with ideals, philosophy, psychology, and the need to understand at the intellectual level. How do you express yourself openly or repressed? How can you open to greater self-expression? How do you use your mind — past, present, future thoughts? Again, focus on your energy on the now and speak your truth free of fear.

SIXTH CHAKRA - THIRD EYE - INDIGO

This is the intuitive center, and pertains to visions, intuitive abilities, and symbols. How do you respond to your intuition - with trust (Heart Chakra link), by acting upon your insights (Root Chakra link), by expressing yourself with your voice (Throat Chakra link), by believing in it with your rational mind (Solar Plexus Chakra link)? What are your psychic abilities, how can you open more to them? Are you aware of the presence of a guide? Do you trust your intuition?

SEVENTH CHAKRA - CROWN - VIOLET

This deals with the ability to receive light. Are you open to the connection of your higher self? Are you visionary? Do you enjoy traveling into other realities, receiving spiritual images and ideas? How do you use your imagination?

Color	Musical Note	Chakra (Energy Body) Location/Function/ Behavior	Color's Effect	Problems Treated
Red	C	1st—base of spine creative, sexual and restorative process transmutation	energizes, vitalizes, heats, and promotes circulation; stimulates adrenaline red blood cell production, menstrual flow and sexual power; strengthens willpower and courage	anemia infertility/impotence colds and chills weak menstruation (not in fevers or nervous problems)
Orange	D	2nd—below navel emotional center purification	warms and cheers, frees bodily and emotional tension; aids mentality	lung ailments epilepsy mental problems rheumatism kidney troubles
Yellow	E	3rd—solar plexus thinking (mental) center ambition	inspires and awakens the mind; strengthens the nerves; helps reasoning; aids self control; aids elimination; improves skin; a cerebral and nerve stimulant	stomach troubles indigestion, gas. constipation liver problems. eczema nervous exhaustion

Green	F	4th—heart area sensitivity—feelings compassion/harmony	harmonizes and balances, soothes and restores; a tonic; stimulates the heart; soothes the nerves, brain. heart, and eyes; helps elimination; refreshes	headaches, heart ailments, ulcers, eye problems, nervous conditions
Blue	G	5th—throat area communication self-expression	antiseptic, cooling, sedative; relaxing, and soothing; helps stop bleeding; helps with nutrition and building the skin and body; promotes truth, loyalty, and reliability	all inflammations, throat problems, fevers, infections, burns, spasms, pain, headaches, diarrhea
Indigo	A	6th—pineal (pituitary area) (third eye) perception realization	electric, cooling, astringent; anesthetic effect; builds white blood cells; increases activity of the spleen; depresses heart and nervous system	pneumonia, mental problems, convulsions, eye, ear, and nose problems
Violet	B	7th—crown (top of head) universal consciousness oneness	stimulates spiritual nature and intuition; elevates inspiration; expands divine understanding	mental disorders, neuroses, neuralgia, concussions, cramps, tumors, scalp problems

WHAT A REIKI TREATMENT IS AND DOES

Information For Clients

I.) Reiki Balances And Works On Four Levels Of Existence
    A.) Physical: The Body & Manifested Pain or Disease
    B.) Emotional: What You Are Feeling
    C.) Mental: What You Are Allowing Yourself To Think
    D.) Spiritual: Your Capacity To Love Yourself & Others

II.) Reiki Works On Cause Rather Than The Effect of Dis-Ease
    A.) Treats The Dis-Ease Rather Than The Symptoms
    B.) Reiki Accelerates Healing, Which May Cause Some Initial Discomfort: You May Heal At A Faster Rate
    C.) How Does This Feel?
        1.) You feel very relaxed as the energy flows through your body. Some even fall asleep.
        2.) You may experience Reiki energy as colors or pure love.
        3.) You may feel peaceful or emotional as old patterns surface.

III.) What Do I Do During A Treatment; What Should I Expect?
    A.) Take Off Your Shoes, Watch, And Metal Jewelry, Disable Cell Phone/Pager
    B.) You Should Relax And Enjoy The Treatment, However Talking Or Asking Questions Is An Individual Matter
    C.) Allow Your Mental Mind To Release All Thoughts & Fears So You Can Focus On The Present Experience, Silence is Suggested
    D.) A Reiki Practitioner Works With The Chakras Or Areas of Specific Pain. There Is No Need For Touching Where It Might Not Be Appreciated.
    E.) A Pillow Is Placed Under Your Neck Or Knees If You Want (This Helps Take Pressure Off The Spine)
    F.) A Tissue Is Placed Over Your Eyes So You Focus Inward
    G.) Enjoy Soft, Relaxing Music
    H.) You May Experience A Shift In Consciousness, This Is An Important Part Of Healing

IV.) After The Treatment?
    A.) Your Aura Is Swept, Front And Back
    B.) Some Feel Energized, Others Feel Incredible Peace
    C.) You Might Drink Eight Glasses of Pure Water A Day For A Minimum of Three Days; This Flushes Toxins Out Of The System. Water Is Important To The Body
    D.) According To The Practitioner, You May Be Advised To Schedule Another Appointment To Maintain Well-ness
    E.) Ask About Absentee Healing
    F.) In The Case Of Dis-Ease, You May Wish To Examine Your Lifestyle And Make Positive, Healthful Modifications

CHAKRA METAPHYSICS
IN HEALINGS

Our chakras are our connection to this universe. The Sanskrit word, "chakra," means disk...these disks of energy are vortices that extend out from the central nerves of the spinal column. These are the major seven axis chakras. We actually have over 88,000 total.

Psychologically, our chakras relate to areas of our lives...starting at the top, there is the spiritual center, the intuitive center, communication, love, power, creativity and survival or soul's purpose issues. A chakra can be restricted by the activities of self or others. By living in the Third Dimension, we are subject to all forms of duality that can create problems for our chakra system. An unhealthy chakra system means an unhealthy body, mind, emotional upheavals, or spiritual crisis. Often the damage to the chakra system can begin in early childhood. A child who is abused, or whose need for love and nurturing are not met, can shut down the associating chakras, the power center or the heart center, for example. The pain of not having a satisfying love relationship in later years may cause us to close down the heart chakra. If one chakra is shut down completely, often times others will overwork to make up for the deficiency of the other. Eventually the strain of over-work can cause each one to malfunction one by one if the stress continues unchecked.

Balancing and healing the major axis chakras can be done effectively, as I have suggested, through a combination of Reiki and meditation. I suggest that you work with your chakras as often as possible, but at least once a week. By balancing these disks of energy, you can maintain balance and health in the physical body, which flows over into the emotional, spiritual, and mental bodies as well. (There are chakras in the etheric field as well!) Just as no person is an island alone, the same holds true to the interdependent chakra system. One sad chakra generally affects another. By attending to well-ness, there is no door, no weak link, for dis-ease to enter the system.

SPINNING CHAKRAS

We can utilize a pendulum, stone, or a crystal on a light chain (length of chain should be five inches minimum) to test the chakras of clients when we are doing Reiki treatments. The client is lying on their back. Begin at the Crown Chakra, pulling in to about eight inches away from the middle, top of the head. If the chakra is open and functioning as it should, it will spin in a clockwise fashion with a diameter of about four to eight inches. If the spin is oval, in a straight line, or less than three inches, you will have to do some extra energy work (explained later) to clear and open that chakra, or any others where needed. You proceed to the Third Eye center (Ajna Center), pulling the pendulum in toward the brow but about three inches above it. Almost magnetically, the pendulum will stop when you have hit the outside of this and all other chakra vortices. At the Throat Center, be sure that the head is back sufficiently to allow for that center to reveal itself, and allow enough room above the chin for the pendulum to spin. Continue down to the Heart Center, the Solar Plexus (just above the naval), the Sacral Center (just below the naval), and then the Root Center, which can be tested mid-thigh, between the legs. The knees are minor chakras which may be tested, but don't be surprised if they spin counter-clockwise, as they generally do.

It is not advisable for you to test your own chakras, as you need a positive and a negative charge for this process to be effective.

* Chakra spinning counter clockwise: If all others are spinning clockwise, then use the symbol for mental clearing and the power key, and press into the confused center. Then set the other hand over it crossed. Then recheck.

* Chakra spinning oval instead of round: Place left hand on body at base of chakra. Extend right hand out and down, position is lower than left hand. ("Pain Drain" to clear chakra) Then sweep chakra in a spiraling motion upward. Shake hands off. Repeat two more times. Recheck.

* Chakra inactive or pendulum motion vertical: This

type of activity generally involves two chakras; the Throat and the Solar Plexus are the most common pair. You must first balance the pair by utilizing the Power Key symbol over the chakra highest on the body. Press it in. Then do the same on the lower chakra. Press it in. Place right hand on higher chakra, left hand on lower chakra for approximately three minutes. Sweep both in a spiral upward (together) three times, shaking off hands in between. Recheck.

* You may involve the client if you wish in this clearing process by asking them to visualize a magnetic net of gold light pulling through each chakra, pulling out any inessential energies. Have them shake the net, transmuting any negativity to light. You might have the client explore the particular chakra for energies or things that belong to others. Ask them to clear the chakra by opening a door and send those energies back where they belong. Then call back their own energy to fill that space.

* If Power boost is needed: to increase the diameter of the chakra, you may ask the client to "find the generator or power source" of that chakra. Tell them they have an etheric wrench to fix the generator so the power gets stronger and stronger.

* Discuss the reasons for dysfunctional chakras: Ask the client if they feel that they are not allowed to express opinions (Throat), or if they feel powerless in relationships(Solar Plexus). This could be from conditions that were created earlier in life.

* Always sweep and clear with love and light.

Reiki METABOLIC PATH

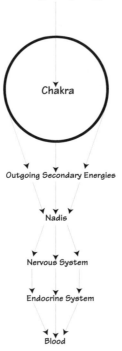

Incoming Primary Energy

Chakra

Outgoing Secondary Energies

Nadis

Nervous System

Endocrine System

Blood

MAJOR CHAKRAS AND THE AREA OF THE BODY THEY NOURISH

CHAKRA	# OF SMALL VORTICES	ENDOCRINE GLAND	AREA OF BODY GOVERNED
#7 Crown	972 Violet-White	Pineal	Upper brain, Right eye
#6 Head	96 Indigo	Pituitary	Lower brain, Left eye, Ears, Nose, Nervous system
#5 Throat	16 Blue	Thyroid	Bronchial and vocal apparatus, Lungs, Alimentary canal
#4 Heart	12 Green	Thymus	Heart, Blood, Vagus nerve, Circulatory system
#3 Solar Plexus	10 Yellow	Pancreas	Stomach, Liver, Gall bladder, Nervous system
#2 Sacral	6 Orange	Gonads	Reproductive system
#1 Base	4 Red	Adrenals	Spinal column, Kidneys

A Torch in Daylight by Reiki Master Karyn K. Mitchell

SELF TREATMENT

People are always shocked when I tell them that I do self-treatment in the car, in a crowd, or during seminars. Almost any time is the perfect time for self-treatment with Reiki. A LITTLE REIKI IS BETTER THAN NONE. Keep that in mind when treating yourself, especially in time of accident, stress, headache, or crisis of any kind. You have this special gift, a tool that empowers you. Use it!

It is important to get into a daily routine of doing Self Treatment. I suggest fifteen to twenty minutes as a minimum to consider. If, for example, you have trouble with insomnia, I suggest that you give yourself a treatment lying down, at bedtime. It is easier to fall asleep with your Reiki energies flowing through you. Other times that fit into your schedule may be just before rising in the morning, as a boost, while watching television, or while reading. If there are other Reiki Practitioners in your home, you may trade "Quick Treatments" with each other, but I still suggest as part of enhancing self-love, that you honor yourself with a self-yreatment daily. This affirms that you are worthy of love and keeps you close and connected to the Universal Life Force.

Some people take Reiki for the sole purpose of maintaining personal good health. This is why Master Takata desired to learn Reiki. She had many physical problems, and she wanted to remain well after her healing treatments in Hayashi's Clinic. There is absolutely nothing wrong about taking Reiki for learning Self Healing techniques. It is, in fact, the first order of business. You heal yourself first, and then you can direct your energies to others.

The procedures that you use for Self Treatment must be comfortable and pleasing to you. I suggest the following techniques until you develop your own method. I do want to mention that in Reiki II, you can utilize the Absentee Method of healing, even with yourself; you can make yourself tiny and place yourself in a cylinder of light that you hold between your palms, or you may treat your back or spine in Absentia by directing the energy through your body to the back. (Your palms are facing the spine, yet held a few inches away from the front of the body.) Any hard-to-reach area of the self can be treated with the Absentee Method.

SELF TREATMENT CONSIDERATIONS

Note: Be sure to treat any part of the body that needs it!

1.) Begin at the head, either at each side above ears,
       or forehead and occipital ridge (headaches)
2.) Throat front and back
3.) Heart Center
4.) Chest (Breasts)
5.) Solar Plexus and Sacral Center
6.) Liver, Kidneys, Ovaries, Intestines
7.) Root Chakra both sides of hips or sit on hands
8.) Knees, Ankles, and Feet
9.) Elbows, Eyes
10.) Hands (By cupping one over the other)

The ideal treatment is three to five minutes on each position, but this may be modified to fit your time parameters. You can visualize that you are treating each chakra with its own healing color:

CROWN: PURPLE
THIRD EYE: INDIGO (BLUE/PURPLE)
THROAT: BLUE
HEART: EMERALD
SOLAR PLEXUS: YELLOW
SACRAL: ORANGE
ROOT: RED

You may also send loving thoughts to each area as you work with it. Share your gratitude for the important work that these parts of the self do for you each day. We suggest that you perform Self Treatment every day following each Reiki Class.

There are two types of Self Treatment. There is what I call Self Treatment Meditation, which may be taken in silence or with gentle music for about fifteen minutes daily. There are also valuable opportunities here and there during the course of the day when you may simply rest your hands where you feel they may be useful for a healing dose of energy. You might apply such quick spot treatments almost any place any time, especially in emergency situations.

the Reiki Boost

by: Master-Teacher Karyn Mitchell

The purpose of the **Reiki Boost** is to provide a quick, energy-lifting vibrational shift in the auric field. This can be accomplished in a very short time, depending on the time that you have to spend on the procedure.

As is said, a little **Reiki** is better than none. In this **Boost** you do not have to place your hands directly on the individual, but can remain in the auric field, just beyond the body itself.

the Reiki Boost

1. Client is sideways in front of you
2. Establish an energy connection by placing both hands on the shoulder
3. Place hands, palms facing nearly 8" apart, just above the Crown Chakra
4. Hold this and each following position for 2-5 minutes or more
5. Palms facing each other go down to Third Eye, one hand in front & the other in the back of head
6. Same procedure, go down to Throat Center, hands front and back
7. Front (one hand) and back (one hand) of Heart Center
8. Same with Solar Plexus, just above the naval
9. Same with Sacral Chakra, just below the naval
10. Treat the Root Chakra, just above the knees
11. Turn palms upward, and slowly lift energy, as you come above the crown, touch little fingers
12. Pull hands apart and sweep aura with the back of the hands as you quickly go down again to knees
13. Snap or close fingers to break energy connection

The Reiki Boost

Hand Positions Part I

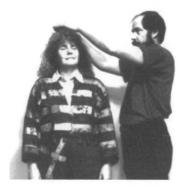

← Begin above the Crown

Ajna Center →

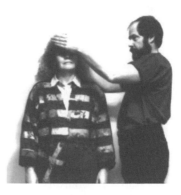

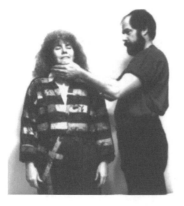

← Throat Center

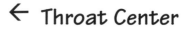

Heart Center →

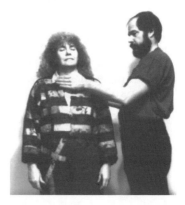

A Torch in Daylight by **Reiki Master Karyn K. Mitchell**

The Reiki Boost
Hand Positions Part II

Solar Plexus →

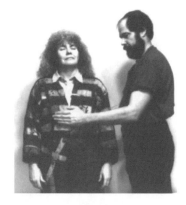

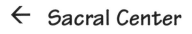

← Sacral Center

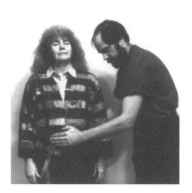

Root Center →

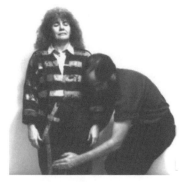

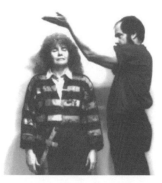

← Up Energy

Quick Treatment

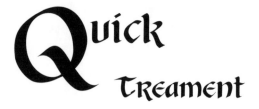

Y ou might find yourself in a situation one day
where you would like to give someone Reiki but
cannot, because there simply isn't enough time, or
you may have an elderly person who is not comfortable on a table.

I n all these cases you can resort to a quick form of
treatment which includes all of the most important Reiki positions.

H owever, never give the impression that you are
in a hurry. Simply make use of the time
available to you and remain peaceful. Even a short
treatment can bring about wonderful results.

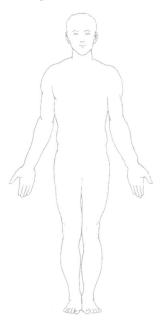

Instructions for
Reiki *Quick Treatment.*

If possible the client should be seated. Start behind the client. Gentle touch, soft knees.

<u>1st position:</u>
Gently lay your hands on your client's shoulders.

<u>2nd position:</u>
Gently lay them on the top of the head.

<u>3rd position:</u> Step to one side.
Lay one hand on the Medulla oblongata (the area between the back of the head and the top of the spine) and the other on the forehead. If they have a headache, ask them to inhale blue and exhale steam several times.

<u>4th position:</u>
Lay one hand on the seventh (protruding) cervical vertebrae and the other in the pit of the throat.

<u>5th position:</u>
Lay one hand on the upper breastbone and the other on the back at the same height.

<u>6th position:</u>
Lay one hand on the Solar Plexus/Sacral Center (stomach) and the other at the same height on the back.

<u>7th position:</u> Move around to front of client.
Place hands on outside of thighs to treat the root.

<u>Optional: Knees, ankles, hands.</u>

<u>Sweep three times.</u>

Reiki has also proved to be excellent as an additional means of giving first aid in the case of accidents and shock. Here you should immediately lay one hand on the solar plexus and the other on the kidneys (suprarenal glands). Once you have done this, move the second hand to the outer edge of the shoulders.

THE FIRST TIME REIKI TREATMENT
OR
TO BE WELL OR NOT TO BE WELL

When a person comes for a Reiki treatment, he or she may not even know what Reiki is or what it does. In fact, this is typical for most who come for a Reiki Treatment for the first time.

What they may have heard about Reiki is that it is stress-relieving; a feeling of total mental and physical relaxation. From my experience, most come because someone else has told them about Reiki. They may know that they can leave all of their clothes on (except their shoes). I find it unusual when a person comes to Reiki knowing that it is a clothes-on experience, but do not know another thing about what happens after they and their clothes get on the table. At least they are open and trusting about the experience itself.

Once in a great while you may have a person come for a Reiki Treatment who has a chronic illness. The reason that they have come for Reiki is to be healed immediately. This is fine, except for the word "immediately." It is important to inform this client that for Reiki to work, one must have patience. This client also needs to know that they may have to do a little life-altering work for themselves. Reiki works, if the person desires to be healed and is willing to raise their own consciousness to remain well. Just as Master Takata learned, it takes time for the Spiritual, Mental, Emotional, and Physical Bodies to be brought into balance and harmony. There are several theories about the number of Reiki Treatments that it takes to heal various physical problems. One theory emphasizes the need for twenty-one consecutive Reiki treatments for the chronic physical problems. Another theory groups various types of dis-ease and assigns number of treatments (as well as definite areas of the physical body to work with) according to the physical problem. I personally feel that each body will determine the number of treatments required to make it well. Aruvedic Science holds the philosophy that the body is like a river, it is never the same from one day to the next. Each body is not only different from every other body, but it can even differ itself from day to day. Therefore, I do feel that treatment must be on a daily basis if a chronic illness is to be healed. If this is prohibitive, I feel that what a person can allow or afford is what will be. A little Reiki is better than none, but in the case of severe dis-ease, then the closer the treatments until the client becomes well, the better. I also feel that if the physical body has manifested a dis-ease, there was an imbalance somewhere in the way that body was treated. There must be a lifestyle alteration of some sort so that the imbalance does not recur. Diet, excercise, and positive thoughts help.

It is our obligation to inform the client of these healing boundaries with Reiki. I also advise that, at this time, you also share with the client that you are merely a channel for the higher energies to flow through. That way they do not begin to see you as a magical elf, but rather as one who has chosen to be such a channel. It is all right to use Hayashi's example of radio waves in explaining the way that Reiki flows through you to them. If they are not able to understand and embrace the idea of being healed by "higher energies," then perhaps you need to ask them how they believe they will be healed. Whatever their belief system, Reiki will heal if they have the desire to be well. I have even asked clients if they want to be well or continue on their current path of dis-ease. The answer is not always predictable, but we must honor the decision as it is theirs, not ours. Again, Reiki is not a religion, and people can heal whether they believe in Reiki or not.

REIKI, THE GIFT OF LOVE

"Reiki means Universal Life Energy and we are all composed of this energy. Everyone can use this energy for healing—and I can teach you how!" (Hawayo Takata)

Reiki transformed my life in many powerful, wonderful ways. But before I get into all of this, let me tell you a secret that I have learned from this Energy. Reiki chooses you, you do not consciously choose it. Many people who are drawn to study Reiki have never heard of it before, and are not really sure what it is or what it does for a person. When I saw the word "Reiki," I knew that it was what I had been searching for most of my life. But I still was not sure exactly what that Reiki was. After my first and second class of Reiki, I still was not sure, but I knew that subtle changes were occurring in my consciousness. When I became a Reiki Master, and later a teacher, I knew that I had received a truly great gift from the Universe, a gift of LOVE.

For over forty years I had lived in fear and had experienced all of its relative emotions...insecurity, separation, anger, worry, illness, low self-esteem, just as many people do. After Reiki, I experienced a new kind of perspective in my life, and this perspective involved living in the now. "Just for today," which is the beginning of the Reiki Principles, means that you define your life to focus on the present. Not the past, not the future, but the present, is what really, truly exists. And if you are not living in the present, you are probably living in fear instead of love. "If...and then..." living is not really living in the true sense, it is merely projecting imaginary thoughts. There is a sense of power in living in the present, a sense of balance, an expanded sense of living in complete love energy.

Reiki is not a religion but a healing connection. It is a healing connection to the Universal Life Force, and therefore a connection to all life, including the self. Healing the self empowers you to accept full responsibility for intending to manifest wellness and joy in your life, and this allows you to empower others to do the same. A true healer is one who gently guides others to self-healing; acting merely as a channel or facilitator for love and light to flow through. "Reiki is One. We are each a part of that Oneness. Be open to this possibility and Reiki will guide you to your Teacher." (Reiki, Hawayo Takata's Story, By Helen J. Haberly)

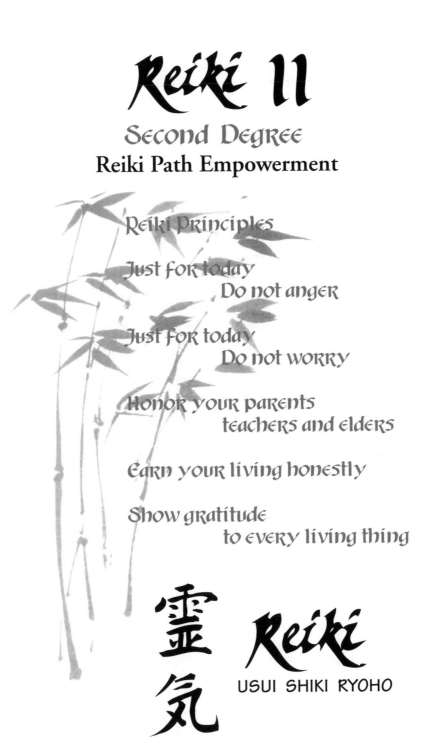

Reiki II
Second Degree
Reiki Path Empowerment

Reiki Principles

Just for today
    Do not anger

Just for today
    Do not worry

Honor your parents
    teachers and elders

Earn your living honestly

Show gratitude
    to every living thing

霊
気

Reiki

USUI SHIKI RYOHO

Symbols

Symbol: "1. Something that represents something else by association, or convention; especially a material used to represent something invisible. 2. A printed or written sign used to represent an operation, element, quantity, quality, or relation, as in mathematics or music." From the Greek word, sumbolon, token for identification. (The American Heritage Dictionary of the English Language)

In second degree Reiki, the student is generally introduced to three of the four Usui Symbols utilized in the Usui Shiki Ryoho, The Usui School of Natural Healing, School of Reiki. The symbols that are shared are the ones that the individual Reiki Master was taught by their Reiki Master. In this fashion, the symbols are shared as a generational experience, passed as the torch from generation to generation. And how are these sacred symbols passed to the next generation? It is different than it used to be. In the earlier teachings, the symbols were what you might call an oral tradition, of sorts. The symbols were shared in class, from Master to student, but all paper evidence of the symbols was burned in a ceremony before the student could leave the room. The student had to demonstrate proficiency in drawing the symbols before they could leave the sanctum of the teaching arena. That is one of the reasons why it was a longer process in learning Reiki, as the student had to know the symbols before they were allowed to depart. Students were oftentimes tested concerning their knowledge of Reiki as well as the symbols themselves.

Some traditions in Reiki honor this ancient method of teaching the sacred symbols. Others now share with their students the symbols on paper. They are allowed to leave with them, generally with the admonishment that the sacred symbols must be honored, revered, and placed in a place where others, who are not Reiki, will not view them. This is the way that I was taught, and this is the way that I teach. That is why you will not find any symbols in any of my books on the open market. I was taught that the symbols should not be out there for just anyone, as they are considered sacred. However, I am also very aware of two very powerful truths concerning the Reiki Symbols: 1.) The Reiki Symbols cannot be used by anyone who has not been empowered to use them, via a Reiki attunement by a living Master in your presence and 2.) The Reiki Symbols, like Reiki itself can only be used for GOOD.

Second Degree Reiki
a Channel for
Absentee Healing, Symbols

I always advise First Degree Reiki students that it is best for them to consider the commitment for Second Degree Reiki before even taking the First Degree. While the hands are a warm and vital part of a practitioner's work, they are not fully functional until Second Degree Reiki Class when they are attuned. The Heart Chakra allows Reiki energy to flow down the arms to the hands after First Degree Reiki, but in Second Degree the chakras in the palm of each hand, which are in the top 40 chakras in the body, are attuned. These then are used to "plug in" directly to the chakra system of the healee. In some traditions of Reiki, only one hand is attuned.

Second Degree Reiki creates a quantum leap in intuitive aware-ness. The energy from the First Degree Attunement is squared, and we begin to make a closer connection to that part of us that was unable to fit into this physical body, the Higher Self. More of the Higher Self Consciousness is allowed to integrate with us. As Master Usui instructed, one must raise the consciousness in order for complete healing to oc-cur. In much the same way, as your consciousness is raised, you may find that your lifestyle changes as well. You may find that suddenly you are making better choices about what you eat and drink. Hopefully you are drinking at least six glasses of pure water a day, avoiding junk food, excess protien, and sodas. Your body is the temple of the soul, where the soul is housed, and it is difficult for a beautiful, spiritual soul or spirit to exist in a not-so-well kept home. At times you may feel that you are on the top of the world, at other times, you may feel sad for no apparent reason. This is part of the clearing pattern that occurs again; that twenty-one day cleansing or clearing cycle that brings up old issues and emotions for you to deal with once and for all. Please read the pages on the Twenty-One Day Clearing Cycle. (Page 28)

Again, it is important to embrace this process; it is like a check mark, you must descend to raise your consciousness to even higher levels than it was before. Author Stephen Levine describes what we might experience during this process:

"Letting go of our suffering is the hardest work we will ever do. It is also the most fruitful. To heal means to meet ourselves in a new way—in the newness of each moment where all is possible and nothing is limited to the old; our holding released, our grasping seen with little surprise or judgement."

After the clearing process comes more personal power and peace. Following the Second Degree Attunement, you will learn how to become a channel for Absentee Healing. This is a process, involving symbols that you are taught. You will learn three of the four Usui System Symbols in Second Degree Reiki. You will be introduced to the powerful Master Symbol in Third Degree Reiki, called the Master Class, when you become an attuned Master. The process of Absentee Healing has been commonly misunderstood. We do not send Reiki energy to one being healed at a distance. We merely allow ourselves to be a channel for the Reiki energies to flow through us to be drawn by the healee. We are not senders of the energy, we are merely directors of that energy. We draw the symbols, focus upon the one to receive the energy (or a picture or a name), and then we allow the Reiki energies to flow through our hands to the healee. The energy is the same as hands-on healing, as the transmission can be compared to talking on the phone. The major difference is that the healee is not experiencing what is called Vitamin T, or the touch of the hands on the body, which allows for powerful endorphins in the body of the healee to be released. In a shorter time span, you will feel that your healing transmission is complete; the general rule of thumb is that fifteen minutes of absentee is comparable to nearly an hour of hands-on work. You should also remember to do absentee self-healing work on yourself for the areas of your body that are difficult to reach. I do this for my spine and lower back.

I encourage students to keep a Healing and a Dream Journal following Second Degree Reiki Class. Dreams can be a powerful bridge between the conscious and the subconscious mind, as well as a link to the Higher Self. It is as the poet Kahlil Gibran stated, "Trust the dreams for in them is hidden the gate to eternity." Some people experience powerful teaching or healing dreams, where it is revealed to them how they can further enhance their spiritual growth. Others may have past life dreams that are apparent because of the antique quality or appearance of the furniture or clothing, or the knowing that the person in the dream does not look like you, yet the personality is the same. Reiki transcends time and allows healing to take place on all levels and all dimensions of existence. Reiki can even heal past lives. Edgar Cayce said, "For life is continuous and whether it is manifested in materiality or in other realms of consciousness, it is one the same."

Reiki II ATTUNEMENT PROCEDURE

meditation:

Prior to the Reiki II initiation, you will be guided in a meditation that prepares you spiritually to become a channel for the higher Reiki energies. During the course of this meditation, you may have the opportunity to meet your personal spiritual guides.

Your Physical, Mental, Emotional, and Spiritual bodies are cleansed during the meditation, etherically.

We may also begin to work with your chakras, starting with the 1st (Root), 2nd (Sacral), 3rd (Solar Plexus), 4th (Heart Chakra, but not the heart itself), 5th (Throat), 6th (Pineal, Third Eye, or Eye of Shiva), 7th (Crown).

initiation process:

Your chairs are placed in a circle with the backs toward the middle. This is to create a mirror effect and will facilitate in creating a greater connection to the energies. You will close your eyes and put yourself in a meditative state. I will place my hands on your shoulders to connect with you and place energy above your Crown and tap you on the shoulder. I ask that you lift your hands in palms touching position above and in front of your forehead. I will blow these energies across your Crown and then clap them into your hands. Then I will lift and align your chakras.

Next I do the same in each hand. I clap each of your hands then I will go behind you to lift and align your chakras once again.

Energy is shared down the spine and then I tap your shoulder and blow through the hands across the Crown. Finally, I place my hands on the occipital ridge and lift and balance your chakras.

Please remain in a meditative state until all have shared the initiation process. When the bell rings, you may open your eyes and join hands in a circle facing the center.

We anchor the energies.

You have now been empowered with the gift of Reiki II.

Please note: Attunement procedures differ among Masters and lineages.

ABSENTEE HEALING
TECHNIQUES

In the Second Degree Reiki Class, you are empowered with the energies that allow you to become a channel for Absentee Healing. This doorway is opened in you through the initiation procedure that connects you to a symbol in Reiki for Absentee Healing. Whenever you wish to open that door to connect to a person or event at a distance, you must unlock that door with the symbol(s) that act as a key to open the way through space and time. We connect with the image or name of the event or person, draw our symbols as you were taught, and then allow the energies to flow through us toward our intention. Again, Reiki can only be used in Divine Order for the highest good, so we must not become ego-involved with the outcome of our efforts. Fifteen minutes of absentee work is worth an hour of hands-on work, and the energy exchange for your services is entirely up to you.

How many ways can you perform Absentee Healing? Is there a "right or wrong" technique? I always qualify that it is YOUR INTENTION that is the most important consideration. Through our network of sharing information and innovative techniques, we have created quite a spectrum of Absentee methods:

1.) The right thigh is the front of the body, the knee is the head, assign body parts as you continue up the leg. The left leg is the back of the body, the knee is the back of the head. You can focus on a full body treatment, or treat only the part of the body that you have time to focus upon. This technique is the most widely-accepted method of Absentee Healing.
2.) You connect to the image or name of the person or event, then extend your palms facing away from you, directing the energies outward.
3.) Visualize a cylinder of light between your palms and place the healee in the center of it. As the hands draw closer and touch, the treatment is complete. A variation of this method is to make a cup of the hands and gently rock (as in the case of a child) the individual.
4.) Do a Reiki Boost absentee.
5.) See the healee on a table before you, and proceed as if you were doing a modified shorter table treatment.
6.) For a burst of healing energy to clear an airplane, hotel room, and transmute energies into light, utilize the Rune Master arm placement. Left palm up to Heaven, arm locked in position, right arm facing out at ninety degree angle from body. (palm flat out).
7.) Place a list of names beneath a candle, crystal, or clear glass or bowl of water. Direct the energies into the list, with the intention that the

A Torch in Daylight by Reiki Master Karyn K. Mitchell

energies are separated by the water, smoke, or crystal. A variation of this is to hold the list between the palms of the hand or hold a box with names.

8.) "Shower" the healee with healing light or water as you direct your energies to them, or wrap them in healing light or bandages.

9.) Petition for the help of a Master, Angel, or Healer to go to the physical place and body of the healee and do hands on healing. See and feel this being done, and it is so. You may go also.

10.) Create a Bridge of Light for gentle, loving support for those who are making their transition. The way is prepared for them.

Absentee Healing has the SAME ENERGY and POWER of hands-on healing. If you call a person on the telephone, the words or power of your words does not diminish or change just because you are not physically there. Trust.

Perhaps the greatest gift of Absentee Healing is the feeling that we are not helpless in times of need and crisis. I would like to relate a couple of incidents where the Absentia Method of healing was gratefully utilized. A Master-Teacher called to relate that her husband had suffered a heart attack on the job. He was being transported to the hospital, and her son was on the team of paramedics who came to transport him to the hospital. "I had almost twenty minutes before I could even leave for the hospital," she relates, "and I wanted to throw myself on the floor and cry. I felt so helpless. Then I remembered to do Absentee Reiki. My son said that he not only felt the energy when it started, but that it had a immediate calming effect, almost as if he had the sense that a great peace had settled in. Her husband's blood pressure began to drop, and the paramedics and doctors could not believe the positive change by the time he reached the hospital!"

Another account: "We got the news that my aunt in (another state) was in bad shape. Even though I was just Reiki Level I, I knew that in Reiki II, I would learn how to do Absentee Healing. I knew it could be done, but I wasn't sure how. I asked my guides, and one showed me how to work on my aunt just as if she were in front of me. I did, trusting that it would work, and I know that it did. It certainly made me feel like I was helping her even though I couldn't be there in person. Now I use Absentee Healing every night for just about everything. I even use it when I see something on the news, like the earthquake in California." What this account brings home to me is the idea of faith. If the healee desires to be healed, does it matter how it is accomplished if our thoughts and intentions are pure? I know that there are many who do not believe this, but I feel that even in Reiki Level 1 we can connect to a Master Healer or Angel who can carry our love and intention over the miles. I mention this in Level I.

Before leaving this space concerning Absentee Healing, I wish to pose other questions for you, the magnificant healing channel. Was the method of Absentee Healing founded divinely inspired by Master Usui, or did it evolve into the realm of Reiki as the need was felt? Was the symbol for Absentee Healing initially for that purpose, or was its original intention for general healing?

Must the body of the practitioner be aligned and straight; in other words, legs and arms uncrossed, or are these body parts like circuits that change the course of the energy? Again, test this energy yourself before committing to an answer.

Is it possible to send Reiki energies into the past to change what is perceived as the future or the present? In other words, can we send Reiki through time for healing? If we leave all work "in Divine Order for the Highest Good," is it appropriate to change our own or another's history? What effect would this have on Karma? Do you believe, as I do, that all time occurs simultaneously.

I encourage all Reiki Practitioners to keep a healing journal like the one on the next page for Absentia work.

We know a businessman who maintains a computerized healing list as well as separate color-coded Absentia lists. The red list is for emergency situations, the green list is for everyday concerns, and the blue list is for people who are dear to him that he sends energy to every day. The lists are laminated and he writes with an erasable marking pen.

ABSENTEE HEALING JOURNAL

"I leave all work in divine order for the highest good, for love, peace, healing, joy and happiness!"

NAME or EVENT	DATE	SYMBOLS USED	COMMENTS

"As Above, so Below, may the healing continue. Thank you for all who helped in this process."

Reiki Absentee Healing Techniques

1. Draw the symbol for the power key.
2. Draw the symbol for Absentee Healing.
3. Visualize the person, place, or situation.
    If you do not personally know the person, speak the name three times.
4. Connect with your compassionate heart.
5. Hold your palms outward so the energies may be drawn by the healee.
6. If the Reiki Energy, is rejected, it is either placed in a bubble for later use, or it comes back to you!

Other Methods

1. Make the person tiny and hold them between the palms of your hands which are held about six inches apart.
2. Place a list of names beneath a glass or clear bowl of water (or a candle, crystal, or pyramid) send your intent to the list by aiming your palms at the list.
3. Rune Master: place left arm, palm up in the air. Right arm is extended, palm out.
4. Assign your thigh the aspects of the body to be treated. Do hands on treatment to your thigh.
5. See the person on a Ɽɛíɾí table right before you and work on the body as if it was there for you.

There are two beliefs concerning permission to perform Absentia Healing. One belief is that it is unnecessary to ask an individual, event or situation for permission as it may prove difficult to do so. In such a case, the Universe or Higher Self of the individual may choose to accept or reject your efforts. Another belief is that Absentia Healing should be requested or permission granted by the individual. We suggest that you follow your own Master's teachings concerning this issue of permission.

SENDING REIKI INTO THE FUTURE

A Healing Message For Planet Earth
by Master Karyn Mitchell

As you may already know, Reiki transcends what we on the Earth Plane choose to call Linear Time. We have the capacity with Reiki to send positive energy ahead to what we would call future events. If you are aware of an upcoming event, you can send Reiki healing energy, love or higher vibrations to that event, or even to a person in the future. That person could be you, or someone that you love.

As always, please leave all healing of this nature in Divine Order for the Highest Good. We create our own reality, but what is best for us is not always best for someone else. However, if we send positive energies forward, they do impact the future in a positive way.

If you are projecting concern about an event in the future, then you are pulling energy from the past, in other words, you are thinking about what has happened in similar events in the past and projecting them into the future. This creates anxiety. If you allow yourself to live in the NOW and focus your energy on what is happening now, then you have more personal power and awareness to deal with events as they happen. In short, you are choosing to act (in Love) rather than react (in fear). If you act in the now and choose to send love forward to future events, then you diffuse anxiety. It is very much like the Western notion of insurance. The reason for insurance is to insure that you are protected from a certain type of loss. It does not prevent the loss, but it supposes that you will feel at least financially better when it happens. A mental concept, is it not? So for those who wish to embrace this mental concept might consider the idea of sending Reiki ahead to future events to insure that all goes for the highest good. Reiki is love, a Healing Light that works only for good. In acting as a channel for future events, we are bypassing what we call linear time, tapping into All That Is or Will Be.

If you decide to work with the energy of Future Reiki, I would like for you to consider sending Reiki Healing Energy to the future of our dear Planet Earth. Please include, in the energy and thoughts of healing, those persons who are in a position of making power decisions for all of the creatures of the face of the Earth. May our healing vibrations, sent forward to our potential future, help those in power to make all of their toughest decisions from the aspect of love, truth and harmony. The politics of war (there are over thirty-two wars on our Earth at this writing) could become the politics of peace; the abuse of the ecosystem could become one of responsible stewardship and atonement (at-one-ment), and all who suffer from dis-ease could find healing. This is my healing hope for the future of our dear Planet Earth, a living, breathing, sentient organism.

REIKI Healing
Release

by: Karyn Mitchell

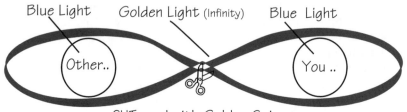

Blue Light   Golden Light (Infinity)   Blue Light

Other..   You ..

CUT cord with Golden Scissors

1. Draw Infinity Symbol before you and press it in.

2. See just the Infinity symbol as a moving, golden Light.

3. Visualize your self in the right golden loop of Infinity.

4. Visualize the one that you wish to release (or past life relationships) in the left golden loop.

5. See the cord that connects the two of you-for instance, if the other manipulates you in your relationship, see the cord running from their Solar Plexus to your Heart Chakra.

6. Cut that cord with golden scissors and burn.

7. Surround yourself in a fence of healing Blue Light.

8. Surround the other in Blue Light until they fade into the distance.

9. Acknowledge that you are FREE.

PRACTITIONERS FOR FOUR LEGGED, WINGED ONES

Reiki for Pets and Animals

PETS

It is my sincere hope that soon there will be clinics and positions in many cities and towns for full-time Reiki Pet Practitioners, a Paws and Claws Reiki Clinic, so to speak. I do know of a veterinarian who does Reiki.

Any Reiki practitioner who has pets or animals at home knows that these special creatures love to be treated with loving, healing, Reiki energy. Once in a great while, you will find a cat who believes that he or she is already so purrrfect that Reiki is non-essential to their well-being. When you work on another human or animal, however, that same cat will be right in the middle of the Reiki treatment soaking up the good energy. It has been my observation that the older the cat or dog the more they seem to appreciate Reiki.

We have used Reiki on all of our pets, and there have been many: cats, dogs, rats, birds, hamsters, and a very spoiled bunny. I would like to be very left-brained and logical about the hand placements for each specific type of animal or bird that you might treat, but it seems redundant to do so since the animal will almost direct most of your hand placements. That is, of course, if you are dealing with a pet larger than the palm of the hand. Please note, however, that surround-

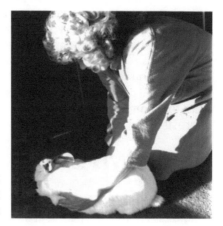

Let the animal guide your hands.

ing a palm-sized animal, like a hamster or mouse, could be too much energy all at once for the poor creature. A sauna in the hands is not always a healing experience. In other words, you could just as effectively treat this tiny creature absentee (if squirmy) or by holding them loosely with one hand above if they will allow this.

Most of our animals fall asleep during their Reiki Treatments, but this is because trust is not an issue with them. If you have a skittish pet that you are dealing with, it may take several sessions in order for them to relax with the energies enough to fall asleep.

Avoid the eyes of most animals in the early stages of treatment, and then treat the eyes later, when they have closed them. That way, they do not panic, fearing that they have gone blind, or in the case of a rabbit, become invisible.

We usually begin our treatment where we know that our pet personalities enjoy it most. For example, our cats seem to like their treatments to begin on the back, just behind the neck. Our bunny prefers that we begin with one hand on each side of her. Our dog likes us to begin on the collar line around his neck. Decide, through experience, where to begin if you have the opportunity to do multiple treatments on your pet. Allow plenty of room for the treatment, and it is always best if you go to them, rather than pull them into your space.

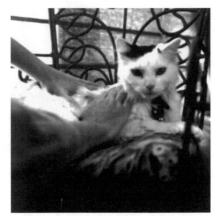

Someday maybe there will be a Paws, Claws & Feathers Reiki Clinic!

No table is necessary in most cases for Pet Reiki Treatments.

If you have fish, you can place your hands on the aquarium glass to direct Reiki energies, or you can sit comfortably nearby and do absentee work for them. Holding the fish in your hands would not be in their best interests.

WILD AND DOMESTIC ANIMALS

Once in awhile a bird hits one of our windows and lies stunned in the grass. We run out, pick the bird up, and gently begin treating the stunned bird with Reiki. Generally, within fifteen minutes, the bird will fluff feathers and fly away. It is also possible to treat birds and wild animals with absentee Reiki if you feel that it would be better for you or the creature that it be done so.

One day I found a small bunny on the road that had been hit by a car. I brought it home and we all took turns of fifteen minutes each treating the little one. It seemed hopeless at first, but after forty-five minutes, it exploded out of our hands, running across the floor. We returned it to the tall grass near the place where I had found it. Please use caution in attempting to treat injured wild animals, however, as some may feel obligated to bite out of fear for their lives. If the animal is in a safe place, be content to do Absentee Healing for as long as possible. Remember, a little Reiki is better than none.

Since we live in a rural area, I make it a practice to send Reiki healing to cows, pigs, geese, chickens, goats and even a pair of ostriches nearby. All animals are worthy of being considered a candidate for Reiki. Perhaps if you

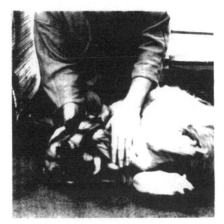

Most animals Love Reiki!

see animals in transit, please think to send them your calming love and Reiki energies to soothe their fears.

ANIMALS PROVE THAT REIKI HEALING IS NOT DEPENDENT ON ANY BELIEF SYSTEM. Animals live in the NOW, in a state of what most of us could consider calling perfect bliss. If an animal is injured or develops physical problems, Reiki can help them to heal. Since they already live in a state of what we could call pure perfect consciousness, it is easier for them to integrate the energies for healing. They make no judgments about the outcome of the treatment, they just accept the energies with gratitude and love.

REIKI AND PESTS

Let me first share with you my thoughts about the word, pest. Animals or insects are not aware that they are in unwanted territory, making your life miserable. We are in their world. What I have done is based on work by the Findhorn Institute in Scotland. A technique that they have pioneered is to communicate with all creatures, great and small, in order to live in harmony with them. For example, when they planted a garden, a row or two extra was delegated for nature's creatures to munch upon. They were informed that this was their space, that they were willing to share their abundance. Few people realize that the Shaker communities in the United States did likewise.

This was, as Eileen Caddy, founder of Findhorn Community viewed it, honoring the "Christ Nature" in all of life. Their creation spirituality was expressed by David Spangler in the forward to Eileen Caddy's book entitled, *The Dawn of Change:*

> *"Findhorn is based on the realisation that the Earth and all humanity are entering a new age, a new cycle of evolution. This change is characterized by several factors, chief of which is the development and manifestation of a new awareness, a new consciousness within humanity which will in turn lead to new patterns of perception and behavior, and to the creation of a planetary culture. The seeds of this new consciousness are within each of us, and can be nourished into germination and growth. Many people are experiencing this transformation. It is not limited to any age group, culture, race, or nationality. It is a spiritual trasformation in the broadest sense of that word, transcending religious and dogmatic boundaries. The new age is fundamentally a change of consciousness from one of isolation and separation to one of attunement, communion, and oneness."*

It is possible to communicate with other creatures and animals. I have tried it, and it works. I have also shared this secret with another Reiki Master who had a field mouse come into her house just as winter set in. I explained to her that the mouse (whom she feared intensely) was there to teach her about that fear, and if she would trust that she could ask her uninvited quest to leave, she would. After the first few encounters, she named the mouse "Hermie," and watched as the creature brazenly ran right in front of her, scaring her out of her wits. She talked to Hermie continuously for three days, the length of time that we decided to give Hermie as an ultimatum to find new lodging in the great outdoors. Her more conventional friends and relatives were urging her to set traps.

It was a great relief when Hermie vacated the premises when her three day vacation was up. She decided that the debilitating fear that she experienced with mice in the past no longer affected her in the same way. Not only had she honored the Christ Nature in her pest. but she also saw and cleared a past life in prison where mice crawled on her in her sleep. Hermie helped to bring up this past life pain and to heal it. Even though she was a humble field mouse, Hermie was able to raise the consciousness of this person.

Please consider compromise and communication first in dealing with pests. I guess I have never really defined the boundaries between pest and human. Who is infringing most upon the space of this Earth?

WHOLENESS AND ONENESS
by: Eileen Caddy

As you raise your consciousness you become very sensitive to that whole new world opening up right there within you. You will begin to feel the wholeness and oneness of all life and find yourselves blending into that wholeness and oneness until you know that all is one and there is no separation.

A GRATEFUL HEART
IS A IS A JOYOUS HEART
by: Eileen Caddy

Your eyes will be open to all the beauty and harmony around you, To the wonders of nature. You will see with eyes that really see; you will hear with ears that really hear; you will speak with words of love and understanding.

Every tiny spark of light creates greater light.
Every tiny spark of love creates greater love in the world.
What you are doing is far greater than you realise.
You are generating more light,
love
and power into the world
by your right and positive attitude.

Do it constantly,
do it consciously.

A BRIDGE OF LIGHT

Technique©1993 Karyn Mitchell

The Reiki Energy that connects to the heart center can be used to heal the four bodies that compose humankind: the Physical, the Emotional, the Mental, and the Spiritual. The intrinsic system that connects these bodies is called the Chakra System. It seems to me that we are not a "Spirit in a Physical Body" (an analogy that seems appropriate here is that of a ship in a bottle) but rather the opposite is true. (The bottle is in the ship.) Our spirit is so expansive, so continuous an energy field, that our physical body is actually in our spirit; our aura is actually an extension of our spiritual body that goes beyond the physical. Again, this is my belief. The Chakra System is a means to hold the spirit, to anchor it, to the physical plane, to the physical body, it connects to the body where it must. Most systems support the major seven Chakra theory. These major seven begin at the Root Center (red, 4-petaled lotus flower, opens downward) located at the base of the coccyx (spine), continues up to the Sacral Center (orange, 6 petaled lotus flower that opens forward) below the naval, to the Solar Plexus (yellow, 10 petaled lotus flower that opens forward) above the naval, to the Heart Center (emerald green, 12 petaled lotus, opens forward) not of the heart but centered in the breastbone area, the Throat (blue, 16 petaled lotus flower, opens forward) located between the inner collarbone and the larynx, the Third Eye (blue-violet, 96 petaled lotus, opening forward) between the brows, and the Crown Center (violet purple, 1,000 petaled lotus, opens upwards) at the top of the head. These seven comprise the central vertical axis, that relate to the most important aspects of human existence, each correlating with different mental/spiritual functions. The petals of the blossoms of each chakra are called Nadis, or energy channels through which energy flows like a conduit Into the chakras.

Ancient, traditional writings mention 88,000 chakras, which means that there is a chakra vortex connecting to nearly every part of the physical body. Only forty of these are considered to be extremely significant, including those centered in the palms of the hands. These in the palm of each hand are important to consider in the study and practice of Reiki, as they allow the energy to flow out and connect into the field of another person or object. We use our palm chakras to plug into the chakra system of another for healing. It is, in fact, through or via the chakra system that we can alter the vibrational field around us; we can consciously or unconsciously radiate positive energy out into the environment, changing the environment around us by raising the vibrational frequency. This is a part of the healing practice, a part of what we do as Reiki . The healing transcends the physical realm, and many who share our space are not even aware that they are being showered with a delicate energy healing. Their divine will will ascertain whether or not they will accept this gift of healing, so they are not receiving something that they may not really want. Again, it is difficult to comprehend, but there are some who do not wish to be healed of their dis-ease.

I wish to share with you my feeling, gained through experience, about what happens to the Chakra-Physical Body connection at the time of transition (death). Through an easing of pain process, there is a disconnecting of the chakras to the physical body. One by one, little by little, either through the process that we have come to label aging, or through disease, we release the hold of the chakra system on the physical body. We are, in a sense, untying the tie that binds us to the physical realm. The last to go is the Silver Thread cord or chakra that is found In the temple area. I have seen this snap or break at the moment of transition. Then the soul can be free of the burden of the physical realm and the physical body. We are no longer attached or confined to the realms of the body. In the case of accident or sudden death, the chakras are torn from their connection to the physical body, which may cause soul confusion. There has not been the preparation for vacating the body, and the spirit suddenly finds itself no longer anchored to a physical body.

BUILDING A BRIDGE OF LIGHT

With Reiki, we can build a "Bridge of Light," a path for those who have transcended the physical plane and are in spirit form. I want to relate to you my method of creating such a bridge, but please feel free to work with your own system of belief. This Bridge can be accomplished through the process of Absentee Healing. You may utilize the symbols that you have been taught for the Absentee Channel. Then you hold the picture in your mental mind of that person or the name if you do not know them personally. You create a "Bridge of Light" to the higher realms or their place of highest spiritual development. This bridge helps the spirit to cross over. Your intention is to dissolve confusion, to comfort and calm the soul, and to show that there is a light out of the confusion. It is appropriate to telepathically communicate with this spirit at this time, soothing their fears and actually allowing them to know that they are no longer attached to the physical plane. In the case of sudden departure, they may not even be aware of what has happened to the physical body. Tell them that you have created this beautiful bridge for their way to the light. Use their belief system, if you know it, to allow them comfort. For example, I say that Jesus or Mary is there with them and will help them across the bridge. You may have them see that there are other loved ones or Ascended Masters on the other side of the bridge to guide them. You may also ask, "in divine order for the highest good," if they wish for you to say something to those that they are leaving behind. They may leave more easily if they have the comfort of communicating to someone their forgiveness or asking thereof. Do not worry about this communication process, however, if you are not allowed to receive communication from them. The channel to the physical is sometimes fuzzy, the other way it is not so. They will receive your blessings and comfort. They will see the Bridge of Light that you have created for them. Stay with them until you know that they have completed the crossing to the other side. Give them love, hope, and blessings. Then you can dissolve the channel by pressing your fingers together and giving thanks to those from the Light who helped with this transition process.

Reiki is UNLIMITED, it is love, its power lies in and beyond your belief system. So allow your gift of Reiki to be a Bridge of Light for those you need to find their way back to the Source of the Light. SHANTI.

Reiki III
Third Degree

Reiki Path Empowerment

Reiki Principles

Just for today
>Do not anger

Just for today
>Do not worry

Honor your parents
>teachers and elders

Earn your living honestly

Show gratitude
>to every living thing

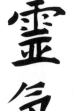 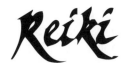

USUI SHIKI RYOHO

Reiki Master
(THIRD DEGREE REIKI)
CLASS

There are different distinctions made in the various traditions of Reiki concerning the Mastership. In our Independent Lineage, the Master Level is attained in the third class, or what some might call Third Degree Reiki. It is in this class that the student receives the Master attunement and techniques and is introduced to the Master Symbol.

Following this attunement, there is another twenty-one day cleansing cycle, cleansing each of the seven axis chakras each day of the week for three weeks. I often have students ask if this is the last clearing cycle. Probably not! From my own experience, I feel grateful that clearing takes place to some extent every time in every way that we choose to utilize Reiki. As long as we are on the Earth Plane we have work to do on ourselves as well as others.

I also feel that part of the work that we must do is to learn to heal with love and humility, as opposed to ego and power. Dr. Elisabeth Kubler Ross has stated in an essay that she wrote called "The Four Pillars Of Healing:"

"In my view there are four essential qualities of a healer: trust, faith, love and humility. The healer must act as a channel--that is, as the conduit of a healing entity or force, whether one calls this God, Christ, the Inner Teacher or whatever. In order to become such a channel, the healer must have absolute trust in its healing power as well as faith that he or she is capable of channeling it. And, although different healers may channel the healing energy by a variety of different techniques, none of them can heal--no matter what their technique--unless they use it with love and humility. Love is perhaps the most problematic of these requirements, because all healers have days when they are not open to love."

So what does the Mastership in Reiki mean for those who aspire to attain it? Your energy is once again squared as it was after the Second Degree Reiki Attunement. However, with the Master Attunement there is a major commitment for service to others. In the broadest sense, we dedicate our lives to become the healing hands of All That Is. Some fulfill this service through extensive Absentee healing work. Others do hands-on healing for individuals or groups with special needs. Some elect to learn the techniques for training others. I strongly suggest that the decision to become a Reiki Master be considered in light of service and example. Not only should you endorse the Five Reiki Principles and the Two Precepts, but you should also choose to live the spirit of Reiki as well. It is much like Gandhi's "Experiments With Truth:"

"The instruments for the quest of truth are as simple as they are difficult. They may appear quite impossible to an arrogant person, and quite possible to an innocent child. The seeker after truth should be humbler than the dust. The world crushes the dust under its feet, but the seeker after truth should so humble themselves that even the dust could crush them. Only then, and not till then, will they have a glimpse of truth." GANDHI, An Autobiography

Mohandas K. Gandhi taught by example. When he was murdered, he left behind a rich legacy of truth and wisdom. His material goods amounted to not quite ten dollars.

I am not expecting you, as a Master, to be a living example who serves on the same level as Gandhi. You must be aware that you must do the best that you possibly can to be a loving channel of these pure Reiki Master energies. You must learn to love even the hardest person in the world to love, and that may just be yourself.

Prior to the Master Attunement, you will learn how to perform the Water Ceremony. If you choose to become a Master-Teacher, you can go on to learn how to attune others (initiate them) in the First Degree, Second Degree and Reiki Master Levels. You must be a living example for your students, and as a Master, you will share with them your unconditional love and support in their progress toward empowerment. When you empower others, you empower yourself. That is a Master's Truth.

Reiki III ATTUNEMENT PROCEDURE

meditation:

Prior to the Reiki Master Initiation, you will be guided in a meditation that prepares you spiritually to become a channel for the intense Reiki Master Energies. During the course of this meditation, you may have the opportunity to meet your personal spiritual guides. These guides may present you, at this time, with your Etheric Master Robe or some other gift that will serve you as the hands of Universal Service.

Your Physical, Mental, Emotional and Spiritual Bodies are etherically cleansed during the meditation.

We will also continue to work with your chakras.. starting with the 1st (Root), 2nd (Sacral), 3rd (Solar Plexus), 4th (Heart Chakra ... but not the heart itself), 5th (Throat), 6th (Pineal, Third Eye, or Eye of Shiva), 7th (Crown).

initiation process:

Your chairs are placed in a circle with the backs toward the middle. This is to create a mirror effect, and will facilitate in creating a greater connection to the energies. You will close your eyes and put yourself in a meditative state. I will place my hands on your shoulders to connect with you. Then, I will direct energies above your crown and tap you on the shoulder. I ask that you lift your hands in palms touching position above and in front of your forehead. I will blow these symbols across your crown and then clap the outside of your hands. Then I will lift and align your chakras.

Next, I do the same with the palm of each hand, blowing and clapping energy into each hand. Then I place both hands back on the heart chakra. Then I will go behind you and lift and align your chakras once again.

Energies are then directed down the spine and blown in to the palms over the head and sealed. Then I lift and align the chakras. After each of the three initiation sites, I will place my hands on your occipital ridge to lift and balance your chakras.

Please remain in a meditative state until all have shared the initiation process. When the bell rings, you may open your eyes and join hands in a circle facing the center to ground and anchor the energies.

You have now been empowered with the gift of Reiki III.

Please note: Attunement procedures differ among Masters and lineages.

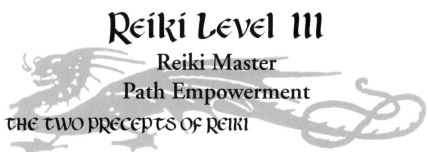

Reiki Level III
Reiki Master
Path Empowerment
The Two Precepts of Reiki

The First Precept:

The person must ask to be treated, and in asking, open the self up at the throat level. They vocalize and say, "I want to change where I am; I want to alter my state of existence." In asking, the person is putting forth a conscious decision to become involved. The request may also be made on the soul level. It is from the Soul level that the person asks for a healing. <u>There must be a change in consciousness for healing to occur.</u> It is essential to listen and render service to the request of the soul.

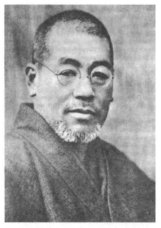

Treat the Cause
not the Effect..

The Second Precept:

There must be <u>an exchange of energy for services</u>, not for healing, The healing energy belongs to the Universe. However, there needs to be a creative exchange from the recipient, the healee, to the person whose time and services are being rendered. An energy exchange can be anything from the stored concept of energy we call money, to an exchange of services between the healee and practitioner. Often we treat loved ones and our family members. If there is an exchange taking place, where one is doing for another consistently, then energy is being exchanged.

Reiki practitioners offering healing services on a professional level do establish a fee. The fee sets a value on the service, which is considered a concrete reality in the thinking of humankind. Wellness, likewise, has a value, and ultimately reflects the feeling of worthiness and self love of the person seeking to change their state of health.

A Torch in Daylight by **Reiki Master Karyn K. Mitchell**   Page 93

HEALING MENTAL DISORDERS
with
REIKI

There are many factors to consider when studying what we might call mental disorders. It seems that nearly one person in one hundred in our Western culture suffers from some sort of depression. In fact, depression might be called the common cold of mental disorders. However, like many other types of mental disorders, depression may occur for many different reasons. Even within the framework of symptoms, what may create chronic or acute depression in one individual (heredity, diet or environment, for example) may not bother another at all. We will first review treating the four bodies with Reiki, including such physical-allopathic aspects as diet and supplements, and then consider the Japanese philosophy of balance and harmony.

Healing the Spiritual Body

THE FIRST BODY TO BE TREATED IN REIKI IS ALWAYS THE SPIRITUAL BODY. The four bodies that we treat in Reiki are the Spiritual, the Mental, the Emotional, and the Physical. In order to gain access to what we call the Mental Body, we must first work with and through the Spiritual Body. Only then do we begin to treat the cause of the dis-ease, not merely the effect or the symptoms.

It is now known that people who are prone to pessimism, sadness, anxiety, and stress are more prone to develop dis-ease. In other words, a poor state of mind can damage health because the brain and immune system work together. A better state of mind helps to create a healthier body. The field of psychoneuroimmunolgy illustrates how the chemicals in the brain influence emotions and our ability to feel pain. The receptors for these chemicals in the brain, called endorphins, impact on both the emotions and the response to white blood cells that attack invading foreign bodies. There is also evidence that natural cancer fighting chemicals in the body, called interleukins, are directly linked to the brain and brain activity. Both meditation and Reiki affect the main cause of disease by working through what psychology chooses to call the psyche, or the human mind as spirit. Other psychological terms for psyche are: anima, soul, subconscious, inner self, pneuma, inner self, or Higher Consciousness.

Einstein's General and Special Theories of Relativity have perhaps brought science or physics closer to a more relevant definition of what spirit actually is. Subatomic matter is actually energy, it seems, that has condensed. This etheric matter acts as a holographic energy template or blueprint that guides the physical body. I feel that when a spirit is subconsciously ready to take on physical form, it works with subatomic particles in order to create this template. Nobel Prize winning physicist David Bohm has created a hierarchy for what he has labeled the Holographic Universe. In the framework of this universe, this hierarchy fits into the order of space and matter/energy. The entire universe is interconnected within the framework of this hologram. This interconnected-ness is All That Is, and by breaking off a part of this and individualizing, we are still a part of the greater whole, only smaller (spirit), yet a part of All That Is. Our etheric body is then our Higher Consciousness or spirit manifested in a physical form. It is as if we are an integral part of an energy soup, if you can visualize that. For the higher energies to be able to flow through to the individual, there has to be a connection or open-ness to the Higher Consciousness.

When Reiki begins to work on this Higher Consciousness or what we call the Spiritual Body, it calms the nervous system and opens the system up to be able to integrate the higher energies that are essential for the healing flow of Reiki energies. It is challenging for an individual to heal if she/he is not spiritually in tune with the higher energies first.

Healing the Mental/Physical With Food

While we are considering the field of psychoneuroimmunology, there are other related considerations in dealing with mental disorders that we need to consider. Diet has been closely linked to many mental disorders, and while Reiki can heal mental disorders, if the individual falls back into old patterns of poor dietary habits or abusive physical behaviors then this leads them back to the same old path of dis-ease. Nutritional deficiencies can cause brain imbalances that result in everything from fatigue and forgetfulness to depression and anxiety. While the brain weighs about three pounds (less than 2% of our total body weight), it uses about 20% of the body's total energy supply. In 1968, a man named Linus Pauling discovered what he called the brain-blood barrier. There may be adequate nutrients for the rest of the body tissues and organs, but these nutrients may not cross the brain-blood-barrier into the brain. There has to be a sufficient increase in nutrients in order to cross over this barrier and supply the brain with what it needs to be healthy. Recent theory holds that the following additional nutrients (most of which are amino acids) are needed to nourish the brain: Ginko Biloba, Glutamine, Tyrosine, Taurine and Methionine, Zinc, B complex (B6 in particular), Magnesium, and Manganese.

Trace minerals are so lacking in the American diet, because of depleted soils, that a growing number of children are suffering Attention Deficit Disorders (ADD) simply because their brain cannot complete necessary synaptic activity for lack of catecholamines, amino acids, or simple trace minerals found in most organic, raw vegetables. Brain waves are transmitted one cell at a time passing to the tip of the axon across the space that separates one cell from another (a synapse) to the receiving cell called a dendrite. The diet derived elements that allow this space to be bridged are called neurotransmitters: adrenaline (produced by amino acids phenylalanine, effective here is DL-phenylalanine, and tyrosine) and serotonin (whose precursor is the amino acid tryptophan). Relay activity continues until the message within the brain reaches its destination, or until it is stopped by lack of a bridge (serotonin). The brain cannot function well if the bridge is not there. Proper diet including trace minerals and amino acids can complete the bridge an allow the brain to function as it should.

Depression may be the result of the body's inability to process lactose found in such dairy products as milk, butter and cheese. It is not uncommon for a person to be placed on a drug called "Prozac" for what is diagnosed as a chronic depression; while this depression may in fact be diet-related. Food allergies or eating a poor quality of food may also be difficult to discern, but may also result in depression.

It is unfortunate that many people know more or care more about the octane of the gas that they use in their car than the quality or ingredients of the food that they put into their mouth. This is why individual consciousness must be raised; we must be responsible for our own physical maintenance. If a person is not willing to take full responsibility for the well-being and loving, nurturing, care of the physical body, then dis-ease will be an obvious consequence of ignorance or lack of caring. That is why we must desire to change, to know how to take care of ourselves, and to love ourselves enough to do so. It is the first of Master Mikao Usui's precepts: "I want to change where I am; I want to alter my state of existence." The person suffering from anxiety, depression, or other mental disorders must be prepared for change on all levels, but first on what we call the soul or spiritual level. She/he must first be in tune with the higher energies before the healing can continue to flow on to the Mental Body.

Healing the Mental Body

When the Mental Body Level is accessed, then, the calmness accompanies a growing sense of well-being and serenity. Balancing can begin on the mental level, bringing with it clarity, dissolving depression and mental confusion. Old patterns may be brought to light and examined through a series of treatments; there may be what seems a worsening of conditions, but this is only part of the releasing or letting go of old toxic behaviors that created chaos on the mental plane. As the old patterns are crystallized, released and swept away by the individual, a sense of well being and self-esteem may begin to take hold. Everything that you think and feel has a direct effect upon who you actually are. If you are always focusing mental or emotional attention upon the past, then you are not really living in the present, in the NOW. The past is gone, and the future is unrealized, so to focus much mental or emotional energy on either actually creates disharmony. Reiki encourages us to live in the now: "Just for today" is an intrinsic part of the Principles of Reiki. By mentally focusing on the present, we are focusing on the true self. An emotion is a thought linked to a sensation; sensation takes place in the present. However, with the help of thought, we have a myriad of experiences in the past. We also have an arsenal of fear that we can project into the future of uncertainty. We have these reference points that we can refer back to in order to respond to a sensation. If for example, the sensation that we are exposed to is pain, then from the memory of that stimulus in the past, we manifest anger. (I am angry because I knew that breed of dog might bite.) In the present, this pain may be experienced as a sense of being hurt. (Ouch, the dog bit me.) Pain projected to the future is manifested in the present as anxiety. (The dog bit me, what if he has rabies?) The energies of this pain can be directed inward and create depression if not eased in an appropriate manner. (This really hurts, I am angry at myself for allowing it to happen, and I might get rabies because I was so stupid. Now I am depressed!) In order to heal on the mental-emotional level of being, we must attempt to respond, and teach others to respond, to all sensations from a level of higher consciousness to transmute bad experiences. By living at all, we are vulnerable to hurt. By living in the now, however, and by bringing in the light of higher consciousness awareness, we can alter our response to one that is more healing. I'm sure that you have heard that we cannot change how someone acts, but we can change our reaction to that person. By choosing, on the mental-emotional-spiritual level how to react to negative feelings or hurt, we can release the painful grip of hurt upon us. We can change consciously and evolve. We can choose to tell how someone or something makes us feel in the framework of the present and then let go of it. We mentally choose not to force hurt further on into the physical level to later manifest as a dis-ease. We are choosing how to change our response to our environ-ment. We are choosing to be well and live in the present. We can say to ourselves: "Just for today, I choose to be happy and healthy."

The conscious choice or desire for change has created a ripple effect through the system of the individual, and is now in the master control center of the body, the brain. The brain has embraced the now and is choosing to be well.

We have also mentioned the physical/chemical aspect of the brain function, but are now considering the responses brought about by the stimulus for appropriate healing: this conscious choice allows for growth, tissue repair, motor functions, digestion, and more empowering physi-cal and emotional responses.

Healing The Emotional Body

When this is the case, then, healing begins on the Emotional Body level. Anxiety, fear, and stress are released, and depression is relieved even further. Anger, resentment, hostility, and jealousy are replaced by more of a feeling of acceptance (not resignation) and trust. This, then, can become unconditional positive regard, or love. The most difficult person to learn to love is the self. We are our own worst critics, always focusing on what is wrong about us rather than what is right. Perhaps this critical voice comes from childhood memories, echoes from the past of someone else who crushed your self esteem. In healing the emotional body, we must learn to affirm our divinity, our all-rightness. We must transcend our past and learn to say to ourselves, "I love and accept myself just the way I am. I am a reflection, an important part of All That Is. I forgive myself of all past mistakes, and realize that in living in a state of higher consciousness, I am replacing previous shortcom-ings with present good acts." In other words, we must shift the critical-ness of the past into an accepting loving present. Our emotional bod-ies need to heal, and we are now empowered with Reiki energies to claim our divine birthright, our right to be loved.

When we love and accept ourselves, then we are in a position to share this love, in a healing intention with others. The emotion of love is the key to all healing. It is the link to All That Is, to all that we are. We need to redefine ourselves to heal our emotional body. Only then can the focus of pain shift: loving, healing, Reiki energy may circulate back to the Physical Body, where headaches or physical pain may be eased. Love, on the emotional-physical level of healing can create a harmonizing within the pituitary and pineal glands and make the healing on all levels of existence more complete.

Mental Disorders As Japanese Ki Stagnation

In considering mental disorders from the Japanese point of view, the focus is a direct result of Ki stagnation. Poor Ki circulation brings impaired actions, thoughts and dis-ease. Insomnia, mental disturbance of any kind, as well as dis-eases of the nervous system are all manifestations of Ki dis-ease; an imbalance or disharmony between Yin and Yang. The Japanese word for dis-ease is "byoki," which translates in our language "the evil of Ki." In later Oriental medicine, dis-ease, is subdivided into categories of "Ki dis-ease," water dis-ease and blood dis-ease. Dis-eases within each of these categories may be either Yin (female) or Yang (male). Yang dis-eases are the easiest to cure. The easiest to treat are blood dis-eases (Yang) because at the end of the digestive process, the food becomes blood. If we eat animal protein for food, then the blood will be too thick (Yang), this creates a desire for sugar, and then the blood becomes too thin (Yin). Both create mental disorders in the body. Again, we are back at the consideration of food as mental medicine.

According to Oriental medicine, Ki disease or mental disorders may also be related to liver problems. I have also heard that anger comes from or is stored in the liver. This is why Master Takata always spent extra time on what she called "the Big Motor" area of the mid to lower body, where most of the internal organs are stored. The liver, the largest gland in the body, has many functions: to purify the blood, release blood glucose as needed, to synthesize or store vitamins, and to create bile that aids in digestion of fats. It detoxifies the body and aids in metabolism. The liver is located in the right, upper part of the abdomen, and crosses over the midline of the abdomen above the stomach. In treating someone with Reiki for what the Japanese would call Ki dis-ease, then, the practitioner might want to focus physical treatment on the anatomical part of the body where their liver resides.

The Use of Symbols, Chakra Balancing

There is an Usui symbol, learned in Second Degree Reiki, that helps specifically to clear mental blockages and will aid in integration. You can add power to this by adding yet another symbol to increase the strength and depth before and after using the symbol to clear mental blockages. Generally these would be used around the head, but you could also use them in the liver area as well. Balancing the chakras at the same time would further enhance healing efforts of the mental/physical/spiritual/emotional level. Pay particular attention to revitalizing and balancing the solar plexus chakra, as mental disorders may be the result of a feeling of a loss of power, resulting in a feeling of despair or hopelessness.

Please remember that the best defense against dis-ease of any kind in Reiki is to achieve and maintain a sense of well-being. Share with your clients your personal philosophies about self-healing with Reiki, or at least allow them to know that if they come to you for Reiki Treatments and Chakra Balancing when they are well, then there is no need for disharmony or depression to set in. In other words, you must educate them concerning their own personal responsibility in maintaining a healthy mind, body, and spirit. Reiki is also sharing with them unconditional positive regard, also known as love. Where there is a lack of love from self or others, there is a feeling of separateness, a sense of loss that penetrates all levels of being. By living in the Light of Love, we are sharing our connectedness, our integration into All That Is. By allowing Reiki to flow through us, we help others on all levels to experience this integration, this Love. Perhaps it is the first time in their life that they have ever experienced Unconditional Love. It is the first step in the true healing of self.

WHAT THE EMOTIONAL BODY IS AND DOES

The Emotional Body functions as a liaison between the Physical and Mental Bodies and the Spiritual. Unfortunately, many in our Western Culture have dis-connected from the Emotional Body in order to function in our socioeconomic culture. This dis-connection can be a root cause of eventual disease in the physical plane, whether it is recognized as depression, stress, or the Monday morning flu. The denial or suppression of the emotions can lodge in the physical body and manifest in the form of illness that can even threaten physical existence.

Emotions serve a great purpose as an expression of the Life Force. These emotions can be channeled into productive forces for self-expression. Expression of the self tends to pull a person from the control of the mass consciousness, and this is viewed as a threat to corporate mentality. In order to be truly healthy, we must learn to transcend emotional barriers and allow our self-expression to flow in creative channels. All emotions teach us about ourselves, about our sacred spiritual nature. We need to feel in order to BE, in order to be alive and vital. Our emotional pain as well as joy and love can teach us what we need to learn, to know about our reality. It can teach us how to experience our boundaries in the physical and create balance, so that we can live in the power of the NOW in the power of LOVE.

The progression of healing begins with the Spiritual Body, to the Emotional Body, to the Mental Body consciousness in each cell, and then to the Physical System that we have created out of our experiences. If we are dis-connected from our Emotional Body, part of the healing process in Reiki is to aid in the integration or re-connection of the Emotional Body. This is why the attunements or treatments in Reiki can cause such disturbance in the emotions of some individuals; they have perhaps been forcibly disconnected from their Emotional Body, and the re-connection can be considered a painful process. It is a healing process and should be honored as such.

In our society, there is too much emphasis on the silver bullet or the quick fix. If you have been allowing disharmony in your life for years and years, it takes a bit longer for Reiki to work, to heal. You must have the consciousness that allows for patience, for integration of the healing energies. Reiki works to heal the cause, rather than the symptoms of any dis-ease, whether it is Emotional-Spiritual dis-connection, or a liver (or Live-R, showing how important this organ/endocrine gland is to the physical body) disease. For every year that an individual has suffered a disease, it takes about one month of healing.

The emotional upheavals that are so apparent in the healing processes in our Western Culture must be embraced and we grow spiritually as a result. This is why the Inner Child work of John Bradshaw has been so effective. We must learn how to re-connect to the Emotional Body, to nurture and love and honor our Self, that part of us that connects us to All That Is. Allow yourself to feel, to play, to Be. You are, as the saying goes, a human be-ing, not a human do-ing.

The Water Ceremony

"Next to the dragon, and connected with it, water is the most frequently employed symbol in Taoism. It is the strength in apparent weakness, the fluidity of life, an also symbolic of the state of coolness of judgment, acceptance and passionlessness, as opposed to the heat of argument, the friction of opposition and the emotion of desire. Water fertilizes, refreshes, and purifies and it is symbolic of gentle persuasion in government of the state and the individual. It occupies the lowest position, yet is the most powerful of forces. The highest goodness is like water. Water is beneficial to all things but does not contend. It stays in places which others despise. Therefore it is near Tao. The weakest things in the world can overmatch the strongest things in the world. Nothing in the world can be compared to water for its weak and yielding nature; yet in attacking the hard and strong nothing proves better than water. For there is no alternative to it. The weak can overcome the strong and the yielding can overcome the hard. This all the world knows but does not practice. This again is the practice of 'wu-wei' and nonviolence. Water may be weak, pliable, fluid, but its action is not one of running away from an obstacle. On the contrary, it gives at the point of resistance, envelops the object and passes on beyond it. Ultimately it will wear down the hardest rock. Water is a more telling symbol than land...crossing the river to get to the other side is, again, attaining the state of enlightenment."

TAOISM the Way of the Mystic by J.C. Cooper

In the Reiki Master class, the student is initiated in the "Water Ceremony." It is important to consider all that water is and does for us, water is life and we are water. In baptizing to new life, water is often the element involved to cleanse and carry the spirit of rebirth. In the Water Ceremony, the breathing technique is used to energize the water, once again, this water is life, and we are this water. What we are doing to this water we are doing, essentially to ourselves and to all of life. We are directing Reiki Energy (the 'Ki,' the vital life force energy that flows through all living things) for wisdom and truth, love, peace and harmony.

WATER some interesting facts to think about.

Water is in dreams and other messages, very symbolic of emotion.
Water is transparent.
Salt water represents grounding of the pure compassionate, love Emotion.
Most of the water covering the earth is salt water. A very small percentage is fresh.
Water has a very high specific heat (stored heat) when compared to other liquids. 2x > Olive Oil, 7x > glass, 30x > mercury.
Water conducts electricity, oil does not.

Hai Ahi Wai The Water Ceremony
Breath-Fire-Water

❖ SITTING IN A CIRCLE, EVERYONE holds A GLASS of WATER *(palms on the sides of the glass, fingertips, but not thumbs, touching).*

❖ Hold THE CUP AT THE SolAR PLExus level.

❖ CONTRACT THE Hui YIN.

❖ THRoUGH your MOUTH, breaTHE WhiTE LiGHT INTO your kidNEys.

❖ ExHAlE forcEfully blue MIST CREATING A blue MIST cloud ABovE your HEAd.

❖ Do THis 3 TIMES.

❖ TAkE IN A breATH of THE blue MIST cloud, hold your breATH, THis ENERGY GOES up your spiNE.

❖ DRAw THE symbol _____ HorizoNTAlly ovER THE cup ANd blow THE breATH ovER THE WATER.

❖ AftER EACH visualizATioN, pass THE cup you ARE holdiNG TO THE pERSON ON your riGHT. WE Now kEEp ouR owN.

❖ REpEAT THE ENTIRE procEduRE 2 MoRE TIMES.

❖ SAy: THE WATER is blue, THE GlAss is blue, THE breATH is blue, THE spiriT is blue.

❖ DRAw THE symbol _____ HorizoNTAlly ovER THE cup ANd slowly dRiNk All of THE WATER.

❖ This ExERcisE will cHANGE THE molEculAR vibRATioN of THE WATER, soME- TIMES impARTiNG A sliGHTly diffERENT TAsTE TO THE WATER. If you cHoosE, fRESH lEMON juicE MAy bE AddEd TO THE WATER. LEMoN WATER HElps TO cuT THE MucUS iN THE sysTEM, ANd Adds ElEcTRolyTEs wHicH ENHANcE THE subTlE ENERGY flow.

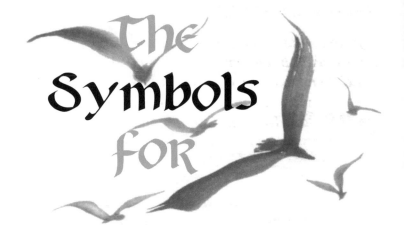

The Symbols for

These symbols were surrounded by the colors of white, blue, purple, and gold. These symbols form the base for the Usui System of Natural Healing. However, only three of these symbols are suggested for use in the art of healing. The fourth is suggested for use only by Reiki Masters. These traditional symbols are to be honored and kept sacred. Other symbols have come through various other healing traditions and may be offered in Reiki classes. Please remember that in Reiki there are only four that are traditional, and you should be advised if others are shared.

Two things surprise me concerning the original Usui symbols. First, that some seem to have survived in what must be very close to the original form, and second, that others are so different in the various traditions. Perhaps the ceremonial burning of the paper that the sacred symbols were drawn on created the drastic difference among these symbols. Passing on the symbols was nearly an oral tradition. Also, I was told that Takata taught her Masters the very same symbols, but through time and various memories, they often were changed. I share symbols with my students in the same form that they were passed down to me by my Reiki Master.

Karyn Mitchell, Reiki Master Teacher

靈

氣

Reiki

The Usui System

Empowerment

Vibrational Frequency Before $\mathcal{R}$eiki

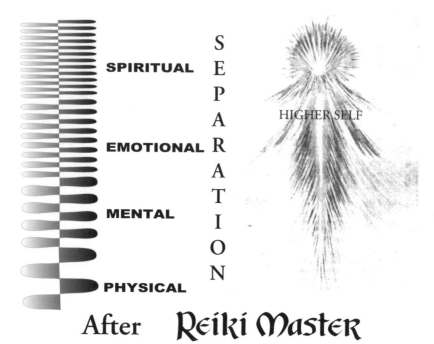

SPIRITUAL

EMOTIONAL

MENTAL

PHYSICAL

S
E
P
A
R
A
T
I
O
N

HIGHER SELF

After $\mathcal{R}$eiki $\mathcal{M}$aster

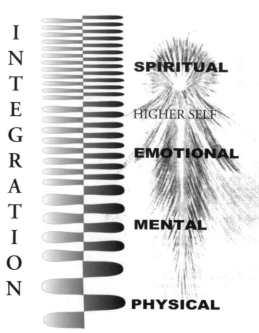

I
N
T
E
G
R
A
T
I
O
N

Reiki Attunements raise the consciousness to allow merging with the higher self energies and awareness. The shift in consciousness allows for greater intuition and balance to occur in the physical plane.

SPIRITUAL

HIGHER SELF

EMOTIONAL

MENTAL

PHYSICAL

A Torch in Daylight by $\mathcal{R}$eiki $\mathcal{M}$aster $\mathcal{K}$aryn $\mathcal{K}$. $\mathcal{M}$itchell

Reiki
Master Teacher

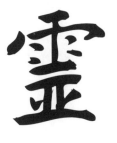

Reiki Path Empowerment

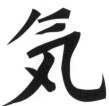

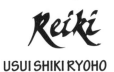

Reiki

USUI SHIKI RYOHO

Reiki Principles

Just for today
 Do not anger

Just for today
 Do not worry

Honor your parents
 teachers and elders

Earn your living honestly

Show gratitude
 to every living thing

Empowerment

by John Randolph Price

I am poised and powerful in the Presence of God.

My emotional nature is quiet, my mind is still, and I am
one with my All-Knowing Self.

Detached from this world, impersonal to illusion, I am
totally open to the Divine Revelations from above.

From the radiance illumination my mind I see only Reality.

From the celestial note issuing forth from the Highest Realm
of my Being, I hear only Harmony.

From the stream of crystal clear essence pouring into my
consciousness from on High, I know only Truth.

From the pure Light of Intuition I know the Way.

I am now able to take direct and correct action.

I know what to do, how to do it, and when.

I am A Divine Knower.

My knowingness now reveals the Plan and my part in it.

I Watch...I Listen...I Wait... I See...I Hear...I Know.

I now move forward to accomplish that which is mine to do.

Dear Reiki Master Teacher,

It has been an honor to serve you as your Reiki Teacher. With great love I welcome you to your new power and responsibility.

Reiki and you are the healing combination that can create miracles. The world needs you both, now!

LOVE, LIGHT and PEACE

Karyn Mitchell, Reiki Master Teacher

WHAT IS A REIKI MASTER?
A MESSAGE FROM THE HEART
by Reiki Master-Teacher Karyn Mitchell

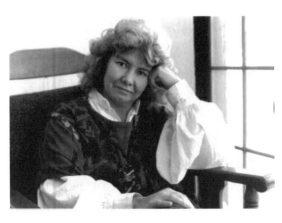

This message does indeed come from my heart, because all that I can really relate to you about What a Reiki Master is must come from there, from what I feel rather than what I Know or can prove on a piece of paper.

I made a personal decision to become a Reiki Master and it changed my life in profound ways. It was from my personal desire to lead the most spiritual existence possible, that I actually made this decision, then created the pathway to achieve what I spiritually desired. I wanted first to be the best that I could be, and then I wanted to share this profound experience with those who desired it for themselves. This is why I teach. Period. Not to gain material success, money, or ego recognition for myself; this is not at all in my consciousness. I choose not to teach my students what they should charge for their services or their classes, but I do suggest that they follow Usui's Precept that they must have an energy exchange of some sort. There must be the exchange appropriate to the respect of the service, one that the client can pay.

Another teaching that I share with my students is never, never,

NEVER, fight about or over Reiki as it is practiced by humanity, on the Earth Planet. It is appropriate to think about the different methods of teaching of Reiki, and to ask questions to advance understanding. It is not appropriate to judge or criticize others who are doing their best to advance the spiritual practice of Reiki. I honor all Masters who are serving the real tradition and the light of Reiki, for the promotion of love and understanding on the planet. I also believe that when the student Is ready, they will find the appropriate master. I am always grateful and heart touched when someone chooses me to be their Master for their work in Reiki. Reiki is taught so many different ways now, that it is more important than ever that you take the time to find a Master who honors the true tradition of Reiki and offers you a strong foundation in the Reiki Trainings. The living Wisdom is important.

There are three aspects that distinguish Reiki from most other healing modalities: Lineage, Self Treatment, and the use of Symbols. <u>Lineage</u>: Reiki depends upon a living Master who shares a hands-on physical attunement with a student, thus sharing their lineage or roots back to Master Mikao Usui. This transmission of lineage must be shared in person, and the Master then teaches the basic trainings in person as well. That is Reiki. <u>Self Healing</u> is a gift of Reiki that is not found in most other systems. Knowing that you are worthy of your own healing is a major focus of Reiki. <u>The Reiki Symbols</u> are an important part of Level Two and the Master teachings as well as empowerment they offer the healing practice. In the tradition of Reiki, these symbols are sacred, and sacred means secret. I feel that those who make their symbols available to others may lose their power much as in the Shamanic tradition where the sharing of the power animal diminishes the power of the animal. Traditional Masters respect these symbols as living energies. They ask that their students hold them sacred as well, honoring Master Usui and his tradition. Respect for energy is truly Reiki. *Namaste!*

WORKING WITH MULTIDIMENSIONAL INSPIRATION:

TEACHERS, GUIDES, AND THE HIGHER SELF

How do we recognize the possibility of spirit or spirit guides when we can not see them in our third dimensional reality? We are taught in our mentally-focused Western Culture that seeing is believing, and if it cannot be seen or explained in a rational, left-brained fashion, it really did not happen or does not exist. This is so enforced throughout our culture that the brain seemingly loses its potential to process intuition or intuitive messages. The more analytical the culture, the more intuition is sacrificed on the altar of the mind. I truly believe that the use of the intuition in life that may or may not result in what we call, psychic, is the allowing or encouragement of such inspiration from early life on. It is easier for such a person to understand and connect to spirit guides, teachers, and the higher self. In contrast to this is one who has devoted a lifetime to analyzing, criticizing, and beating reality into a visible black line. I am not saying that it is impossible for extremely left-brained individuals to connect to intuition or guides. What I truly feel is that they must experience a sort of death of the old self in order for the door to intuition and multidimensional thought to be opened and then the information to be trusted as not only important but credible.

In Mircea Eliade's book, *Shamanism, Archaic Techniques of Ecstasy,* Eliade relates that in some cultures, individuals who relate to spirits for guidance and information, the "region of the sacred inaccessible to other members of the community," are considered the elect of that social structure. They are considered by some to be the "messengers of the celestial god who dwells in the highest sky."

Unfortunately, Western Civilization has thumbed its proverbial nose at Shamanism dismissing both it and a belief in spirit guides as primitive and potentially chaotic. In truth, it cannot be controlled by the society and is therefore viewed as a potential threat to modern cultural definitions. We must be instruments of conformity, not believers in spirit guides or messages.

I like Leo Buscaglia's response to society's tendency to embrace such banal conformity: "If people think you are crazy, they will leave you alone. Then you can do almost anything you want." For some of us who have wasted decades trying to fit in to a rigid social structure, it is a relief to be free and fly once again as we may remember doing in our early childhood. You may have even been bold enough to share your wonderful experience of flying with your angel friends with an adult, only to learn that this is not only impossible but dangerous. "You can't fly and don't you forget it! And never, never, mention your imaginary friends to anyone, they'll take you away and lock you up!" And then, in that brief instant, in the fear that those words might be true, you are bound for the rest of this incarnation to the dirt of this Earth Plane, never to fly again.

Some people need flying lessons, and that is what this is all about. This is "Flying 101," or how I learned to leave my left brain behind and reach for the stars with my soul. In "Seat of the Soul," Gary Zukav states:

"It is natural to ascend to a level where you can learn to distinguish between the sources of guidance that you receive. The idea of being guided by truth that is received intuitively appears unusual to the five-sensory personality. The psychology that has been constructed upon the experiences of the five-sensory personality does not even recognize intuition in the sense that it recognizes, and studies and seeks to understand, physical perception, affect, and cognition. To the multi-sensory personality, it is unusual 'not' to rely upon truths that it receives from its higher self and, through its higher self, from souls that are more advanced. The personality is never separate from its soul, and the soul and its personalities are continually assisted and guided with impersonal compassion and wisdom."

Before the flying lessons, perhaps we should take just a moment to define some of the terms and instruments we will be using. You may already be wondering what Higher Self means. It may come as a surprise to you, but the entirety of the soul does not incarnate in the physical body. The box is too small for the gift, so all of the gift does not come into physical be-ingness. This part of the soul that is beyond the physical body is what we might choose to call the Higher Self. The Higher Self is the soul's method of speaking to the personality that is incarnate in the physical body, and this communication process is what we could label intuition. We must learn to embrace, if we have forgotten, this intuition and trust the guidance. The problem comes when the analytical brain wants to qualify the source of the information. If fear or doubt creeps into the process, the knowledge or information is not honored. It is then polluted by a series of doubts. The most common doubt is, "What if I made this all up myself?" Or worse yet, what if I tell someone this information, and they ask me how I know and they'll think I'm crazy!? Zukav assures us that:

"Higher Self connecting to nonphysical teachers produces a level of truth that is true not just for you, but that would be true for anyone who came into contact with it...Answers that come through your intuitive processes or through intuitive channels may challenge what you would prefer to do. Your lower self, your personality, will not challenge, but rationalize."

Beyond the Higher Self, and with its help, we can connect to guides, masters, and teachers who will help with soul growth. The old sage saying relates that when the student is ready, the teacher will appear. I believe that our non-physical teachers guide us from the moment of incarnation, and are delighted when we are ready to acknowledge that they truly do exist even though we may not see them. It is very much like what Master Jesus said to his disciple, Doubting Thomas, "Have you believed because you have seen me? Blessed are those who have not seen and yet believe." (John 20:29) It is not for these non-physical teachers to tell us what to do. They are not the directors of this play in life that we have chosen. Rather their divine purpose is always to connect us to our soul's path and purpose for being here; it is the job of the teacher to remind us of our own chosen lessons in this life. And they love us, unconditionally, no matter what.

Guides and Masters have specific knowledge that can prove to be useful to us. They are not always with us, but they are there if we will only call upon them for help; we have infinite wisdom at our sincere request. Masters or Ascended Masters are accomplished souls who choose to stay close to the Earth Plane to help advancing souls to achieve enlightenment if that is their wish. Saint Germain, for example, has been labeled the Master of the Aquarian Age. This "Keeper of the Violet Flame" played an instrumental part in the development of the democracy of the United States. In order to truly work with such a Master, one must be reaching sincerely for higher consciousness and desire it enough to alter their existence. Working with Ascended Masters is not always the easiest path to follow, as one must learn to abdicate all notion of fear and embrace totally the notion of love for self and others. Loving self is not selfish, but rather like the oxygen mask that drops from the plane in an emergency; first you must put the mask on yourself, then you can be of service to others.

I have had people ask me if it is possible for a living, breathing, human being to appear to them as a guide. Of course it is. Perhaps your Higher Self knows you better than you think! There must be some element of trust in the physical appearance or wisdom of the guide in order for you to honor the message, however. In Reiki, we are reminded of the story of Takata, where the spirit of Hayashi appeared to her at the foot of her bed. He tells her that she must return to Japan at once, as he is prepared to make his transition. She hops on a boat, journeys to Japan and finds Hayashi standing in his living quarters in perfect health. She said to him, "Why did you send for me?" She did NOT say to him, "I must have been crazy to come here!" Her faith in Hayashi as a Spirit Guide saved the tradition of Reiki. Her trust in the message brought Reiki to all of us.

In Shamanism, teachers and guides appear as animal spirits, as well as in human form. Is it the message or the messenger that is most important? Again, it is a matter of trust and honoring the information that is brought to you for discernment. I always say, run the information through your heart, for it must feel like truth for you to integrate it into your being. The more you learn to trust, the more will flow to you, and the easier the process of connecting to the higher energies will become.

SOUL FLIGHT
Meeting Your Guides
A Guided Meditation

In a quiet space, find yourself at peace. Focus on your breathing, and each time that you exhale, move further back into your inner awareness. Let go of your mental mind just for a short while; give it love and then ask it to be still.

You feel very safe, warm, and protected. You are open for what spirit has to show you. You are ready to meet your guides, masters, teachers, or angels. All you have to do is ask that it be so, and we will embark upon an incredible journey to connect to the love and wisdom that is there waiting for you in the form that you have asked for. For our purposes, in this guided meditation, I will refer to those whom you have desired to meet simply as your guides. You will know, in your heart, who it is that you most want to meet at this time on your spiritual path.

See yourself going back to a time in your life when you were young, innocent, and trusting. You are a child once again, a child on a treasure hunt. The treasure map is right in front of you, and as you gaze upon it, you see that where you start is right where you are. The path that is to lead you to the treasure is just how you picture it. Perhaps it is rocky and dusty, or maybe it is covered with green grass or bark. If you would like, it could even be a yellow brick road. It is your way to the treasure, and in the spirit of childhood adventure, you set out, light in heart and filled with joy. See how bright the sun is! Feel the warmth of that sun penetrating every cell, nerve and fiber of your being; smell the freshness of the day and feel the light breeze blowing through your hair. Feel how good it feels to be you in this expansive, loving place.

As you journey onward, you notice that you are beginning to go upwards. Your path is leading you higher and higher until you feel that you could almost touch the clouds. As you reach out, you grab a cloud that is just the right size for you. You are excited about where this cloud may take you, so you jump onto it, right into the middle, and you snuggle safely down into its fluff just far enough to feel very safe. The cloud soars upward, higher and higher. Then, you notice that the Earth is no longer visible, you see only stars, and the solar system as you see it now, is beyond your ability to describe. You have reached the limits of the Third Dimension, and you feel a slight pressure as you push through the membrane, a membrane that feels very much like cellophane, that separates the Third Dimension from the upper realms. As you break through this layer, it becomes intensely bright and you hear beautiful

A Torch in Daylight by ℞єіκі Master Karyn K. Mitchell

tones and music. You look around you, and as your eyes adjust to the brilliance of this new light, you see that your cloud has landed on a cosmic surface. You step off this cloud and look ahead in the distance. You see shapes approaching you, and you know that these shapes are your guides. Take just a moment and ask that you be allowed to see all of the details that you need in order to understand, ask to feel all that you need to feel, and ask that you have the faith to believe that what you have asked for is being revealed to you at this time. As the guides get closer and closer, you feel their radiant love for you. They are happy to see you, and you notice the smile that is for you alone. "It has been awhile since you've been here..." says your guide telepathically, you sense. It is as if the words from these loving guides are flowing directly into your consciousness, and all of the questions that you have held in your thoughts for so long are being answered without a sound from your lips. You are in humble awe of their wisdom and unconditional love for you. Take all of the time that you need to communicate with your guides. Tell them with your thoughts that you are ready to accept their wisdom and guidance from now on, and that you honor them for helping and loving you.

From this time on, you do not have to journey so far to reach your guides. They can come to you with a simple thought or if you merely whisper their name in your mind three times. It is a great comfort to know how close they are to you at all times. Your guides melt all fear with their love, wisdom, and power. It is your power now, your wisdom, your love...for they are there to share this with you. Thank your guides, and if you are ready, climb back into the center of that fluffy cloud, and gently return to the beginning of your treasure hunt, then back to this room, to this place and time. You have found your treasure much closer to home than you ever imagined, and it is so.

We thank the guides for their help. It is an honor to work with them for the purpose of healing and the sharing of love.

CREATING A TAPE FOR MEDITATION

I suggest that you create your own, personal audio tape by reading slowly from this meditation script. You may change any words or phrases to suit your personality needs. It may also be helpful to play soothing music without words in the background as you create this tape.

You may listen to this tape as many times as needed until you make soul contact with your personal guides. Enjoy the experience!

Reiki Path Empowerment Code of Ethics
©1997 Karyn and Steven Mitchell

• The Code of Ethics of Reiki Path Empowerment is to promote professional standards that protects the integrity of the profession and spiritual practice of Reiki, and safeguards individual clients and students.

 • Those practitioners and teachers of Reiki Path Empowerment in the exercise of professional accountability will:

1. Have a sincere commitment to provide the highest quality of care or education and provide compassion and loving kindness free of prejudice to those who seek their professional services, to practice the Reiki Principles and Precepts.

2. Represent qualifications honestly, including education and professional affiliations, and provide only those services which the client requests and you are qualified to perform. If a client seeks only Reiki, then only pure, traditional Reiki should be practiced. If any other modality is applied, the client/student must be informed and must consent to it.

3. Accurately inform clients/students, and other health care practitioners, as well as the public of the education, experience, and limitations of their training. This includes all advertising, cards, and verbal information.

4. Provide hands-on treatment only when the client personally requests, and allow the client to choose future treatment with no pressure from the Practitioner, as serves their Highest Good.

5. Maintain and improve professional knowledge and competence, striving for improved and loving service through continued education, experience, sharings, and spiritual practices.

6. Conduct business and professional activities with honesty and integrity and respect the inherent worth of all persons, Mother Earth, and her plants, animals, and minerals.

7. Keep a clean, safe place of practice that insures the privacy and comfort of the client/student.

8. Refuse to unjustly discriminate against clients/students or other ethical health-serving professionals.

9. Keep all client/student information confidential unless written permission is given to share with another or others, vital information that

may promote health and well being within the family or the community.

10. Respect the client/student's right to treatment/education with informed and voluntary consent.

11. Respect the client/student's right to refuse, alter, or end treatment.

12. Provide treatment/education in a nurturing manner that ensures the safety, comfort, and privacy of the client/student. Student/client must be informed of hand positions in Reiki, and there is to be no touching of genitals, buttocks, breasts or any private areas of the body unless written consent is given. An example of such a case might include the topical treatment of breast cancer when and only when the client requests and written consent is given.

13. Exercise the right to refuse to teach or treat any person or any part of the body for just and reasonable cause.

14. Refrain always from initiating or engaging in any sexual conduct or speech, sexual activities, or sexual behavior involving a client and/or student even if the client/student attempts to promote such a relationship.

15. Avoid any interest, activity or influence which might be in conflict with the Practitioner's obligation to act in the best interests of the client/student or the profession and spiritual practice of Reiki.

16. Respect the client/student's boundaries with regard to privacy, disclosure, exposure, emotional expression, personal and religious beliefs, and the client/student's reasonable expectations of professional behavior.

The Teachings of Reiki 1
First Degree
Reiki Path Empowerment Class
Reiki 1

The student is introduced to a simple meditation technique in order to prepare for the Reiki I initiation. When the student is ready, there is a transfer of energy that opens you up to a universal energy we call Reiki. You then become a facilitator for channeling healing energy. Hand positions are introduced, as well as the chakra system, visualization, clearing the aura, closing, and ethics. It starts a 21 day cleansing cycle of the 7 major chakras.

Reiki 1 Class Content

SUGGESTED CONTENT FOR CLASS SESSIONS

for Reiki 1:

1)   Two to three hour session - Include history, chakras, principles, precepts, use of energy, meditation, attunement. Vegetarian lunch.

2) Two to three hour session - Instruction and hand placements in Self Healing, Quick Treatment, Reiki Boost, Table Treatment.

3) One hour table treatment. More time is allowed for larger classes. Closing circle.

A Torch in Daylight by Reiki Master Karyn K. Mitchell

The Teachings of Reiki II

Second Degree
Reiki Path Empowerment Class
Absentia Healing

Reiki II

Introduces the symbols that are used for Absentia Healing and symbols to work with such issues such as past-life, karmic, mental healing, and emotional healing. The energy transfer further opens you to the Reiki Energies.

TREAT THE CAUSE NOT THE EFFECT..

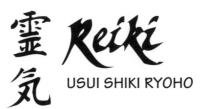

霊
気 *Reiki*

USUI SHIKI RYOHO

Reiki II Class Content

Reiki II Class Sessions Suggestions

1) Two to three hour session - Include instruction, meditation, attunement.

Vegetarian lunch.

2) Two hour session - Include introduction to symbols and practice using them for Absentia Healing. How symbols are used in Absentee, Self Treatment, and in a Table Treatment.

3) One hour healing session for all students. Closing circle.

> *"I never expected my life or my body to ever feel so right, so good. Reiki has brought me profound peace, even in the eye of life's hurricane."* C.H., after Reiki II
>
> *"I had a tumor in my breast shrink from the size of a golf ball to the size of a pea. I expect it to be gone soon, I told my doctor it was Reiki."* K.R., Reiki II Student

The Teachings of Reiki III
Third Degree
Master Empowerment Class

Reiki III   Master Class

Completely opens you to the **Reiki** Energies. It also starts the 21 day cleansing cycle of the 7 chakras. **Reiki** breathing is introduced, as well as new symbols to aid in energy flow from the higher dimensions. You receive the highest traditional attunements as well as instruction and practice in using the Master Symbol that completes the Usui system.

Reiki Treats the Cause not the Effect..

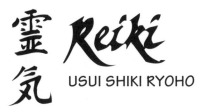

霊
気 *Reiki*
USUI SHIKI RYOHO

Reiki III Master Class Content

Reiki III Master Class Sessions:

1) Two to three hour session - Include meditation, Master Dedication, advanced trainings and techniques, water ceremony, Reiki Master attunement.

Vegetarian lunch

2) Two to three hour session - Include introduction to the Reiki Master symbol, Tonglen meditation, Mental Treatment Methods. Introduction of 18 Beyond Usui System Symbols.

3) One hour session- Vertical Reiki and Nine Nurturing Four Ki Bodies.

Reiki Master Teacher, Class Content:

I WOULD SUGGEST DOING THIS AS A CLASS FOR TWO OR MORE SO YOU CAN OFFER MORE PRACTICE.

1) Two to three hour session - Include Meditation for World Service and teach Reiki I attunement procedure and have student practice and discuss what to cover in Reiki I class.

Vegetarian lunch

2) Two to three hour session - Teach Reiki II & Reiki III attunement procedures and have student practice, teach selected segment, and go over what to cover in Reiki II & Reiki Master classes.

3) One hour session - Review all Reiki attunements, certification requirements and materials.

I always share with Reiki Master Teachers the importance of continuing an active healing practice. Reiki continues to teach us with each experience. Daily Self Healing is extremely important in spiritual evolution as well as for physical well being.

THE MASTER TEACHER CLASS

The decision to embrace the position of Master-Teacher is not an easy one. It is a clear call for service, and should be considered carefully. A Master Teacher has a responsibility to teach the same methods of Usui Shiki Ryoho, The Usui School of Natural Healing, that they were taught, thereby preserving the historic integrity of the tradition and honoring their Master.

The focus of the Master Teacher Class in our tradition is upon techniques of teaching. The Master of that class does not endow you with a personal attunement, but I truly believe that attunements and the practice of attunements create a sense of receiving higher energies, almost as if there is an attunement of a higher order that is shared.

Students are taught how to conduct the attunement procedures for each level or degree in Reiki; this includes the energies that are used at each level. It is important that the student have a working knowledge of the Usui Symbols and how to draw them accurately.

It is also important to insure that each student learn the tools that they need to operate at each level or degree. The following list represents the absolute minimum that should be taught at each level:

I.) First Degree Reiki:
    A.) History
    B.) Meditation
    C.) Attunement
    D.) Self Treatment
    E.) Quick Treatment
    F.) Reiki Boost
    G.) Hand Placements for Table Treatments

II.) Second Degree Reiki:
    A.) Meditation
    B.) Attunement
    C.) Symbols

D.) Techniques For Absentee Healing
E.) Chakra Spinning, Advance Table Techniques
F.) Using Symbols in Table Treatments

III.) Third Degree or Reiki Master
A.) Meditation
B.) Water Ceremony
C.) Introduction to Master Symbol
D.) Attunement To Master Level
E.) Clearing Energy
F.) Tonglen Meditation
G.) Nine Nurturing Four Ki Bodies
H.) Mental Treatment
I.) Vertical Reiki
J.) Introduction to Beyond Usui Symbols

IV.) Master Teacher
A.) Attunement Procedures For Each Level
B.) Attunement Practice For Each Level
C.) What To Teach At Each Level
D.) Materials
E.) Techniques and Meditation
F.) Reiki Sharing/Networking

One question that is often asked in Reiki Classes concerns treating another if you are not feeling well. What I suggest to students is that they must honor the self. If they feel that their degree of wellness allows them to offer a treatment to another, then they may do so. Often a headache will disappear during a Reiki Session. I also encourage students to do daily Self Treatment, especially prior to treating another.

Gathering the Energies Meditation

Following introductions at the beginning of each Reiki Class, we create a circle of intention. Those who can stand do so, keeping the knees soft, and we join hands by placing left palm up for receiving, and right palm down for sending energies through our circle. The intention is set for sharing and clearing energy in the body, mind, and spirit. This also assists with grounding.

May this energy of the Highest Light that we share in this sacred space in this circle be available for all beings in the Universe who need and are receptive to it. In Divine Order may it be.

Take a deep breath and close your eyes. Think peace. And now, with another deep breath, call your energies back to you from wherever they may be, through all of time and space, past present, and future. "Just for today do not anger. Just for today, do not worry." Call your energy back from anyone to whom you may have given your energy, or from anyone who may have taken it from you for any reason. Reclaim your energy. Now, sensing this energy as a color, purify this energy with your breath and bring it back to you where it needs to go. Breathe this energy back into your Spiritual Body and expand your consciousness. Breathe this energy into your Emotional Body and feel compassion for all life. Breathe this energy into your Mental Body and say, "I reflect Divine Wisdom." Breathe this energy into your Physical Body and experience your sacred core. Take a sealing breath of White Light energy and say to yourself, "I honor my life as a gift, I am whole." Feel the integration of this energy through your being.

See a sacred tree before you, the Tree of Life. Merge your consciousness with this tree and feel your roots growing deep into the rich soil of the earth. At the core of Mother Earth, there is a radiant fire. <u>Breathe the fire of Mother Earth into the red of your Root Center, and as you exhale release any energy that is no longer serving your Highest Good.</u> Experience this exhale of release as the color gray or black. (Repeat what is underlined and substitute Root with each of the chakras: Sacral Center, orange; Solar Plexus, yellow; Heart, green; High Heart, turquoise; Throat, blue; Third Eye, indigo (deep blue); Crown, violet. Breathe the fire of Mother Earth into the silver of the Soul Star and the gold of the Tao Centers. As these chakras are purified, breathe the gold of the Tao Center into the Central Meridian. Say, "I am in harmony with the Universe." Open your eyes, hug, and share this harmony.

White Light

White Light (as in healing light-vibrancy) has 2520 electrons, and when run through a prism is refracted into seven primary colors. This calligraph gives off great light vibration, and should be painted exactly as below only much larger and then framed to hang upon the wall of your Sanctuary. We place one in each car.

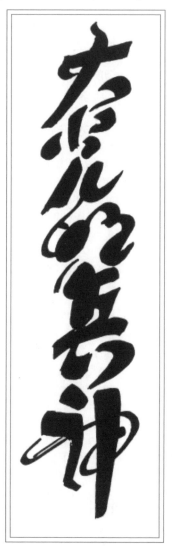

A Torch in Daylight by Reiki Master Karyn K. Mitchell

Reiki Sharing:
SHARING THE LIGHT

Nothing quite compares to the sharing of love energies that a group of Reiki Practitioners can generate. We gather each month with the intention of sharing healing energies with each other and our dear Planet Earth. It is also a time for contemplation, meditation, sharing new ideas and techniques, and allowing the group energies to merge for the purpose of absentee healing. I will briefly explain our Sharing agenda, but encourage you to meet in groups of any size to, as we call the group experience, "Sharing the Light."

Prior to the general Reiki Sharing Group meeting, we hold a short Master Teacher Seminar. The purpose of the Teacher Seminar is to clarify any questions that arise as a result of teaching or practicing Reiki. No matter how attentive you are in class, when you go out into the world as a Master Teacher, there are always questions or concerns that are generated by the teaching experience. One example of a seminar question that was recently brought before the group concerned absentee healing: "Does Absentee Healing work if any part of the practitioner's body (as legs, arms) is crossed? Does it change the energy in any way?" For considerations on this question and innovative techniques from our sharings, refer to the chapter on Absentia Healing.

During the general meetings, we open with guided meditation to bring our energies into the group and help us to focus on integration and self-healing. Also during this meditation, we may bring in, for the purpose of healing, the visual image of one other person.

After the meditation (about 15 minutes), we allow a short time for sharing techniques. At each general meeting, we have a topic to focus on, and the focus is shared with a handout prepared by all who wish to contribute information. Pieces of paper are passed, and we compile a list for absentee healing that is placed beneath a white candle. If there are crystals or stones that sharers wish to place around the candle, this is the perfect time for that. We unite our energies to become a powerful group channel for absentee healing for individuals, events, animals, plants, machinery, and last but of utmost importance, Mother Earth Herself.

The tables are prepared for individual healings. It is our intention that each person who comes to the Reiki Sharing should have (if they desire) the opportunity for a treatment. We share our healings in meditative silence. It is a powerful time of love and committment to healing ourselves and others.

Networking is an interesting side effect of our Reiki Sharings. We meet new practitioners and share information that has the potential to transform our lives. We hold the space for healing to continue in our lives and the lives of all we touch. "As Above, so Below, may the healing continue."

Agenda for Sharing:

Approximate Time Allowed is 2 1/2 Hours
 I.) Master Teacher Sharing Time (30 minutes)
 2.) Reiki (Group) Healing Meditation (15 minutes)
 3.) Sharing Techniques and Handout Information (15 mins)
 4.) Compile Absentee Healing Lists; Place Beneath Candle
 5.) Absentee Healing: Individuals and Planetary (15 mins)
 6.) Individual Table Treatments (75 minutes)

PLEASE NOTE: ALL TABLE TREATMENTS SHOULD BE DONE IN SILENCE TO HONOR ALL PARTICIPANTS.
Remember that our goal is not to draw attention to our ego by telling another what is wrong with them. We encourage wellness with our gentle gathered energies.

REIKI SHARING SHARING THE LIGHT
Absentee Healing

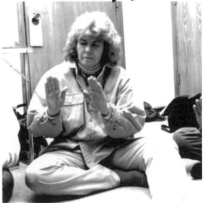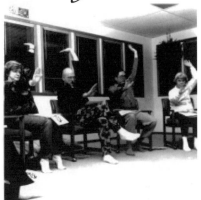

Reiki Boost

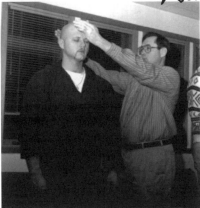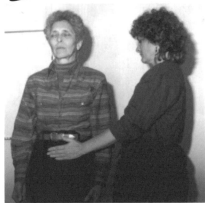

Table Treatments

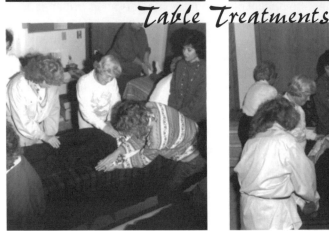

THE IMPORTANCE
OF MEDITATION

Meditation is a powerful, life-altering physiological and psychological tool for change. The Vedic Scriptures teach us that we are not physical beings capable of a spiritual experience, but rather spiritual beings having a physical experience. This explains what happens during meditation:

> "In meditation the active mind is withdrawn to its source: Just as this changing universe had to have a source beyond change, your mind, with all its restless activity, arises from a state of awareness beyond thought, sensation, emotion, desire, and memory. This is a profound personal experience. In the state of timelessness you have the sensation of fullness. In place of change, loss, and decay, there is steadiness and fulfillment. You sense that the infinite is everywhere...Now that meditation has entered the mainstream Western cultural experience, researchers have applied scientific measurements to the subjective experience of silence, fullness, and eternity. In terms of aging, the most significant conclusion is that the hormonal imbalance associated with stress—and known to speed up the aging process—is reversed. It has been established that long-term meditators can have a biological age between five and twelve years younger than their chronological age." By Deepak Chopra M.D.

I have heard students complain that their minds are too busy to be still. What I ask them is, who is in charge of your mind? The Buddhists call it "monkey mind," indicating a lack of personal discipline. The monkey wanders without aim or direction toward an unknown goal. It is part of spiritual development to direct the thoughts toward the highest energies possible. Dr. Chopra says that "the quality of our attention determines what happens to us." Through meditation we can focus on joy, happiness, love, and living in the present, the NOW. We can empty our minds of all that happened to us during the day; to continue to focus on our work or our job is to create even more stress and give more of ourselves away. Meditation helps us to heal stress and take back our own power by claiming peace and happiness rather than perpetually creating stress, anxiety, and fear about the past and the unrealized future.

There are many ways to meditate, many paths to the same spiritual mountain. I am offering as a guide, the guided meditations at the back of this book that I utilize during various class levels of Reiki. That does not mean that you must use these; you may create your own. Just meditate, don't worry about doing it right.

Practice
MEDITATION

Mantra Meditation: Calm your mind. Using a one or two syllable sound as 0m or Shanti, utter these sounds aloud over and over allowing the vibration of the sound to resonate in harmony with your brain and heartbeat.

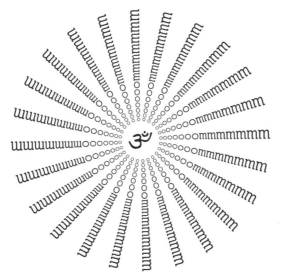

Breath Counting: Focus the mind on the breathing (1-10 count) as it goes in and count out in a slow, steady rhythm. If thoughts enter just acknowledge them and allow them to drift away. Repeat.

Energy Running Meditation: Allow the energy to enter through the crown chakra. Pull it down with the breath to each of the chakras as if you were directing a slow waterfall. Allow the energy to flow down into the ground, or feel it recirculating back up from the crown and back through again, purifying each cycle. You can change the type of energy to cold, hot, or healing. You can also assign the energy a color to correspond with the purpose of the energy bath, for example, blue for healing.

Candle or Aura Meditation: Trakatam. Focus your mind on a candle flame in a darkened room. Soften the rods in your eyes (semi-close eyes) until you can see all of colors of the rainbow. Calm the breath and the mind. Great practice during the bath.

Wisdom of the Vedanta

(self-realization from the "Upanishads")

Meditation

There is a Knowledge beyond knowledge, won only by the brave, who soar on wings of love, beyond the knowing mind. The penetrating laser-light of intellect is able to comprehend the spoken truth — but it cannot know the source of its own light.

It can form myriads of concepts about the knower, but it cannot turn its light on itself and thereby know the knower. To know that knowing self, we must set out blindly, without words, without images; even that shining intellect which is our pride and joy must be left behind.

With no borrowed or reflected light, with no idea-projecting faculty to cast images on the cave-wall of tile conscious mind, we must enter naked, empty-handed, and alone into that dark light.

Without intellect, without a preconceived identity or even existence, unknowing, unseeing, guided only by a faith in truth and the longing of a pure heart, we may enter into the silence of that all-knowing light.

There, no questions rise to separate the knower from the known.

There, the knower is alone — with a knowledge beyond knowledge, won only by the brave, who soar on wings of love, beyond the knowing mind.

by Swami Abhayananda

Reiki and Guided Meditation
A POWERFUL COMBINATION
FOR HEALING

"... all strength, all healing of every nature is the changing of the vibrations from within—the attuning of the divine within the living tissue of a body to Creative Energies. This alone is healing..." (1967-1)

"For the Mind is the Builder—or 'as a man thinketh so is he'—so does that mind, that body, that soul, expand to meet the needs of same." (564-1)

by Edgar Cayce

According to a biological formula, the lifespan of animals should be eight to ten times the age at which it is first capable of reproduction. Humanity, then, should live to be at least 120 years old. If this is so, then modern medical science is not performing adequately in the area of preventing illness and keeping us well. We have more cancer, heart disease, diabetes, mental illness, arthritis, and birth defects than any other industrialized nation in the world. According to one study, Americans rank twenty-first in total life expectancy among industrialized nations. Are you surprised?

There are many things that you can do to help yourself to a vigorous lifestyle and a longer, healthier life. The unfortunate fact remains, that in our society, more time is allocated in education to learning foreign language than in how to treat the body and mind in a nuturing, life-enhancing way. We are never really taught how stress can create havoc in third dimensional bodies, promoting atheriosclerosis and coronary-artery disease.

By utilizing the combined therapies of Reiki and meditation, I believe that stress not only can be brought under control, but avoided entirely. A human be-ing can learn about the proper balance in life, a balance of work, play and meditation. A human do-ing needs to learn (through meditation perhaps) that he/she is really a human be-ing, and needs to focus on the NOW, rather than the past or the improbable future. Sometimes this takes a great amount of effort to convince human do-ings to look inside and decide if they are happy or even content with their lifestyle. Then I teach these humans how to meditate. I tell them that there are several types of meditation, to choose the type that suits them best. I tell them not to worry about doing it right, just worry about doing it. I suggest ten minutes in the morning and ten minutes in the evening for starters. If they are stress-prone in the middle of the day, I also recommend that they take a stress-buster meditation at lunch time. If these people have real "monkey minds" that wander and dart about, sabotaging their efforts, I suggest to them that they utilize one of the relaxation tapes that I have made, or read one of the meditations (on a tape recorder) for relaxation that I have included in this chapter. I have also included a meditation for healing.

If you have had any energy training such as Reiki, I also suggest that, as you meditate, you do self-healing work by placing your hands on the chakras during the meditation. I have included a list of the chakra names and locations in this book.

A guided relaxation meditation with Reiki or other energy work can reduce stress and prolong your life. A healing meditation utilizing Reiki can be created by you for you. Just place your name in the meditation wherever it fits and know that your mind, body, spirit, and emotions will respond to your suggestions. Whatever the mind can conceive and believe, it can achieve..." (Napoleon Hill)

MEDITATION
AS
A FORM OF HEALING

I ask that everyone meditate as a form of self-healing. We are too filled with the importance of busi-ness that we forget the most important connection of all, our connection to the source, to the Universal Life Force.

My goal is to help you to reconnect with spirit in this meditation experience. It is important that you realize that it does not matter whether you meditate right or not, just that you meditate. I have been meditating for over thirty years, and I'm still not sure that I'm doing it right. But that has not stopped me, I still keep trying and enjoying the effect more and more with each attempt. So, let me help you at least get on the path. Please continue on your path, meditate at least once a day for five to ten minutes. A little meditation is always better than none, and the time that you spend is well worth the feeling of renewal that you will experience.

In one Japanese tradition, eighteen minutes is considered an appropriate length of time for meditation. Certain incense sticks provide the experience of an eighteen minute burn, thus eliminating the need for clock watching. When the burning ceases, the proper length of time has elapsed.

In the Zen tradition, the eyes are narrowed but not closed, allowing the meditator to focus upon emptiness. A mudra or hand position is often used in meditation, as the right hand resting on the left in the lap with thumbs touching, symbolizing the union of the Earthly with the Divine.

Becoming All Life
Standing Circle Meditation

©1995 Karyn K. Mitchell

It is a beautiful spring day in the garden of your mind. As you walk through a gentle field, just ahead of you you notice an ancient tree. This is the oldest tree that you have ever seen. The branches of this tree are gnarled, reaching upward like old hands grasping at the sun. The thinner branches are bursting with new leaves to nourish the body of the elder. As you approach the tree you are curious about its life and what it has witnessed. As you breathe out carbon dioxide, the tree breathes it in and transmutes it into oxygen for you to inhale. How many other forms of life depend, as you do, upon this tree and its generations that follow for air, shade, food, and shelter from the night? You touch the rough bark and allow your consciousness to merge with the tree. You feel rooted deep in the soil. So deep are your roots that you can feel the heartbeat of Mother Earth echoing through your trunk. Your leaves are stirred by the gentle wind and bathed in warm sunlight. You are very aware of the cycles and seasons of life. As the rain falls down around you, you move deeper into the roots and follow the rainwater through the depths of the soil.

Allow yourself to become a drop of water flowing underground into a gentle stream which grows into a raging river. You feel yourself crashing against rocks as you are propelled toward the gulf. You merge there with saltwater, flowing out with the water into the deep, cool ocean that knows no sunlight. Drawn by the tides and the mysteries of the moon, you join a wave that washes against the warm sand of the shore. Become the sand for a moment and feel the stillness of a grain of sand resting on a vast beach. You glitter in the sun and are kissed by the tide once again. Become the wave and then the ocean. In your depths, there swims a dolphin. The dolphin plays in the water and leaps high in the air. The other members of your pod are there around you. Moving along the surface of the water, you see a boat. Curious, you approach the boat. There are people with nets aboard the boat. Gain a deep inner sense of how you feel about those people and the net. As you move quickly away, you are playful again, living in the moment. You leap into the air again, breaking the surf. In the sky is a gull.

Allow your consciousness to transfer into the gull drifting on the currents of the wind. The gull feels hunger burning inside and so you fly to the boat. Your experiences in the past have taught you that sometimes a morsel of food may be gained there. Hovering above the boat, a bucket is tossed toward the ocean. You plunge through the cries of the other gulls and win a small morsel. Gliding to the shore, the others like you fight you for that food. Hunger motivates you. You know hunger too well. As you fly off again, you notice a small bunny in the clump of grass where the sand ends. It is new to life and frightened by everything.

Become that bunny awed at first by life but also food for most predators. A child running up the beach frightens you back into the warm, fur-lined fold of your mother's nest. Allow yourself to feel totally safe and nurtured as you snuggle against your mother and rest. When your mother stirs to leave, you follow her out. The first creature that you see is a tall deer grazing in the nearby forest. Allow your consciousness to merge with the deer. Wary of every sound, you run deeper into the forest to join the others of your herd. It is sunset in the forest, and as you bed down for the night, all heads are turned out toward the world in the sleeping circle to protect the elders who no longer smell or hear as acutely. Rising at dawn, a strange scent permeates the forest. It is a man carrying something in his hand that glistens with the sun's rays. Hearts pounding, the herd runs as swiftly as the oldest legs can move through the brush just beyond the ancient tree.

The ancient tree is a witness of life and death. The tree observes in silence as the man moves toward one of its children with a chain saw. The tree has lost many generations to such men. As the man tugs vigorously upon the rope of the chain saw to start its motor, cast your consciousness into the heart of that man. Allow your awakened consciousness to raise the consciousness of all humanity. Think the thought, "all life is one, harm none."

The man sits down in silence beneath the tree. The saw is still and will remain so. He has awakened to the thought that the tree and all life is sacred. His killing has ended. May all of humanity be blessed with the power of kindness and compassion. May the consciousness of humanity be raised in deeper understanding that all living beings contain sentience.

May all beings be loved, may all beings be blessed, may all beings be healed. "SHOW GRATITUDE TO EVERY LIVING THING."

A Reiki I Meditation

Recorded on tape by: Karyn Mitchell 1992

You are relaxed and at ease as you count from 10 down to one with each breath going deeper. In spirit form you realize that you are now walking on this path that is leading up this beautiful mountain. As you are walking, you feel that the path is becoming steeper and more narrow. With every step that you take, you are coming closer and closer to a higher, spiritual space.

Suddenly you realize how heavy your burdens from the past have been. You stop for a moment and notice that the backpack that you are carrying with you is too heavy for your weary shoulders. You take it off and examine the contents of this bag. You notice the first compartment in this bag is labeled "physical burdens." These are negative messages concerning your physical body that no longer serve your highest good. Take a moment and study each of the note cards that contain a negative message about your body. Be aware of the source of this message, and how long you have embraced it. When you are ready to release this negative message and any others concerning your physical body that are present, place that note card beneath your foot. Your body feels lighter as you let go of these old patterns.

The next compartment in your bag contains negative

mental patterns. There are thoughts that you have held in your mind that no longer work for you; these are thoughts or judgments about yourself or others that no longer serve your highest good. This is the place where the inner critical parent resides. Take a look at each negative mental message that is there, and aware of its source, place it beneath your foot if you are ready to let go of it.

The largest compartment contains old emotional baggage. Searching inside, you see that there are things that have created emotional suffering and pain for you in the past. While you have learned from these experiences, you no longer need to drag them or their open wounds with you. Take a look at each emotional burden, and aware of the source, place those cards that you are ready to release beneath your foot.

The last compartment contains spiritual information about you in the past. Spiritual limitations or guilt, shame, and blame may be present here. Forgive yourself and any others that you are willing to forgive and release the cards that prevent you from unconditional love of self and others. As you release and forgive, feel your spirit expand. Say to yourself, "I love and accept myself and other beings."

Now that the backpack is empty, shake it out and observe if there are any hidden messages for you that you need to let go of. If there are, place them and the bag atop the note cards. With the lighter in your pocket, burn all of those things that have limited your spiritual growth. Hear your inner voice say, "I am free!" The flame and smoke transmute all of those old burdens.

You continue your journey feeling light and peaceful. But as the way becomes very steep, you reach a solid rock wall. You know that you may not go a step further without help or guidance. From the space of your own heart, ask that a Guide, Master, or Angel of the Highest Light assist you. As you turn around, you see, sense, or feel an energy coming toward you. If they wish, they may allow you to see their appearance. Notice their eyes, their clothing, their compassion if you can. You may also ask their name simply by questioning, "What is your name? What is your name? What is your name?" If it serves your highest good, a name may be shared with you. They encourage you to place the palm of your hand on the solid rock wall, and it opens to seven golden steps. You ascend these seven steps easily and effort-lessly, knowing that this is a great leap in your spiritual path. 1-2-3-4-5-6-7, and as you step out on the top of the plateau of this mountain, you observe a great cosmic fire. This fire represents the energy and Light of Reiki.

Suddenly there are others there with you — High Spiri-tual Masters who have gone before you or will follow you in the tradition of Reiki. Feel their energy and their love. You feel the warmth of the fire and you join these others in a circle around the fire.

As you are holding hands with each other, you feel the loving energy flowing through you and you experience the smoke and the subtle scent of sage. You realize that you are being purified — that your chakras are being cleansed and purified for this Reiki Initiation on the Spiritual Plane. You feel the red of your Root Chakra being cleansed and purified, it vibrates and opens; moves up to the orange, and you feel the Sacral Center as it is purified. It vibrates and opens. You feel the yellow of the Solar Plexus Chakra being purified, it vibrates and it opens. You feel the emerald green of your sacred Heart Chakra as it is purified, vibrates, and opens. The blue of the Throat Center responds to the energy and is purified. The indigo, or violet blue of the Third Eye Chakra vibrates, opens, and is purified. Finally, the Crown Chakra with its brilliant purple violet, is purified, vibrates and opens wide. All of your bodies are showered with a rainbow of color. You feel your Emotional Body, your Physical Body, your Spiritual Body, and your Mental Body purified. A rainbow of energy is washing through you like a gentle rain, cleansing any energy that does not serve your highest good.

You are prepared to receive the attunement at the Spiritual Level. One of the ancient Masters draws you to a seat before the Reiki Fire. You are brought into harmony with all of the others who are present. This prepares you for the physical attunement that your physical Master will share with you. You allow the energy of Love and Light to become a part of your awareness. In the distance you hear an ancient temple bell as it rings three times. You feel complete.

The Master or Guide or Angel who is closest to you or whose energy you feel the most is handing you a gift, a precious gift that you can bring with you from this high Spiritual Mountain. You are asked at this time in your mind if you are ready to accept Reiki — to accept the Reiki tradition, and the Reiki Principles. If it is your desire to do so, you now accept and acknowledge that this is the Path for you. The gift in the box is for your own healing. Take it out of the box and understand how it may assist you. If you are not certain, ask the one who gave it to you what it is for.

It is time to depart. You show gratitude to those who have assisted you in this process. See yourself descending the seven golden stairs, knowing that you are bringing with you all of the energies that you have received. As you step out onto the mountain path, you notice how vibrant the world is around you. Everything seems fresh and new. Feel yourself once again returning to your physical body, coming back from the mountain, coming slowly back into this room. Begin to feel your fingers, your toes, and when you are ready, and completely back, you may open your eyes. And we will prepare for the Reiki Initiation. Om Namaha Shivaya, I honor the Divine Light within you.

EAGLE MEDITATION
A Reiki II Meditation

Greetings of love, light, peace, joy and hope.

I would like you to begin by taking a long, slow, deep breath, all the way down to your root chakra. As you exhale, tell your body to relax. Take a second long, deep breath, and as you exhale, let go of all of your thoughts and clear your mind. As you take a third long, slow, deep breath, feel your body melting into the earth, becoming one with it. As you exhale, release all of the stressful energy that may be within you at any point and any place.

Feel yourself being nurtured by the earth, by the soil, by the love, that surrounds each and every one of us.

Feel as though you are growing into a beautiful tree. The type of tree is of your choosing, the form that you have in your mind. You become the tree. See your roots going deep, deep down through the soil, pushing gently away at any stones, any insects; gently moving closer to the source of all life. Feel yourself drawing sustenance and nurturing from the soil, from your roots. Feel your arms as limbs as they begin to stretch to the sun. Feel the sun nurturing every part of your being. Your leaves and branches are warmed by the sun. The gentle wind that caresses each and every one of your branches helps you to gain a real sense of what nature is, of what life is. As you are feeling so much a part of life, I want you to see a nest on one of your branches. High up on the top, the nest holds an egg. Suddenly you are the egg and you are choosing to be born again as a beautiful eagle.

See yourself now, emerging from that egg, growing to full form as a powerful, powerful eagle with a wing span of ten feet. Feel the power in your body as you spring from the branch. With your wings outstretched you glide along the air beneath your wings, you are going higher and higher and higher. Through these eyes of yours as an eagle, you see ahead in the distance a spiritual mountain. You are drawn to this mountain, and as you get closer and closer to this spiritual mountain, you see there is a plateau and a tree with a strong limb. You land upon this limb and you wait, looking. Then you see coming towards you, forms of beings. As they get closer, your spirit jumps from the image, the body of the eagle, to the plateau. You are meeting your spirit guides, your masters, perhaps even your twin flame or your guardian angel or angels. You see them as more and more appear, those from the light, that wish to come to help. You are humbled by their power and their love. You feel their love go through you as they take you, one or two of them, by the hand. They lead you to a beautiful, warm, majestic waterfall of many colors. You realize that these are the colors of the rainbow, the rainbow that is within you. You begin by stepping through the mist of the red, and you feel your Root Chakra vibrating open with the power of this red energy. Then you go to the orange, and you feel your second chakra, your Sacral Chakra, vibrating open. Next you step through the yellow mist and you feel your yellow chakra, the Solar Plexus, vibrating open. Then the beautiful emerald green (or pink) that you see as your Heart Chakra and as you step through this mist, you feel your Heart Chakra vibrating open. Then your throat begins to open as you step through the blue, the beautiful blue mist, next you step through to the indigo, the beautiful purple-blue violet that is your Third Eye and you feel this chakra vibrate and open. Then you step through to the purple and then you feel your Crown Chakra vibrate and open wide to your spirituality, and then the white, which is your Soul Star. You feel that vibration above your head and you feel all of these colors showering down around you, awakening your body and your chakras to these beautiful rainbow colors that you are.

Your guides and your masters, and those who have come to help you are in a circle around you. They lead you now to a beautiful fire, very much like a campfire. At the center you see the flames and you focus upon them, as you realize in this meditation that you are a co-creator of your own reality. You begin to make your connection with your masters and your guides and they want to know if you are ready to accept the responsibility, the love, and the healing of all that comes to you now. In showing that you do, in your mind you put your hands toward the fire and you feel the flame against your palms, warm but not burning. You sense that you are part of a group that is so powerful that you can send healing, love, and light to any part of the earth that you desire. While you are in this circle of love, light and flame, you each have a connection with a part of All That Is, with a part of nature, and if your spirit so moves you, you may say something about this connection at this time. We humbly ask that you share with us your thoughts and now leave the spirit with you to speak as you are so guided. We share such thoughts as:

"May the sun forever shine bringing the light of the spirit to those hearts that are searching, those hearts that are open to receive the love that I have to give."

"As the healing energy passes through us, the masters and teachers, we want to share it with one another and with all of our fellow spirits traveling along with us in this life."

"May all be open to the gifts from Mother Earth, the gifts of the native spirits, the Devas, the Light Beings, the rocks, the minerals, the crystals and the flowers. All are gifts for us to be with. May we all feel that oneness and that love."

And now as you rise from the campfire, you embrace in a circle of love with all those who have come to help you, to guide you throughout this physical incarnation and the spirit beyond. You are presented, from two of your closest Masters, a beautiful blanket with symbols on it, and this blanket is for you to realize your power and the power is in love. The power is in healing. The other master or guide presents you with a beautiful feather. The feather is very special to you because it is a symbol of something in your life that needs to be healed or perhaps it is a symbol of a new energy for you, a new power, if you would. You take these gifts with great gratitude and you feel your spirit being drawn into that of the eagle once again and these gifts are held close to the breast of the eagle. Again with the eagle eyes and eagle wings you spring forth from that branch and you soar higher and higher toward the sun realizing that you are one with all of life, there is no separation. As we heal even ourselves, we heal the planet.

You begin to spiral downward toward the earth and you settle gently once again near the nest in the tree and as you quietly breathe, you again become one with the tree, you are again the tree and as you breathe, you feel yourself being drawn back into your own physical body. You feel and sense your fingers and your toes, and you feel your heart remaining open to the gift of love from the masters, and it is so. When you are ready, you may open your eyes. Prakasha and Vimarsha, illumination and awareness are yours.

Reiki MEDITATION
A Reiki III (Master Meditation)
FOR SPIRITUAL ENHANCEMENT

Recorded on tape by Karyn Mitchell 1994

You feel completely warm and protected and at an arms length, you are completely surrounded by a warm, white healing light. You are very comfortable, safe, and you are very warm. As you are sitting there, in this warm healing place, you sense that there is someone standing before you. Your awareness acknowledges that it is one or more than one of your guides who have come to lead you to a special temple. Your guides extend their hands to you and you rise and follow them. As you step forward you realize that you are ascending into the cosmos. You are ascending on a special celestial path strewn with beautiful stars. As you step upwards you follow your guides into what seems to be a soft floor of clouds swirling beneath your feet, and you follow until you come to a great and beautiful door. This door, you realize, stands between you and becoming one with the spiritual advancement that you have been seeking. You raise your arms (as your guides have) in acknowledgment and readiness of this spiritual advancement. The door to this new spiritual kingdom slides open, and you step inside the doorway. Before you lies a beautiful city, a beautiful golden city that draws you closer and closer to it. In the middle of this city you realize that there is a sacred building...a beautiful purple amethyst building and the guides are leading you there. You follow your guides forward into this beautiful place, and as you enter into the doorway notice that there are many, many other guides, many other high spiritual beings who have come to this place to aid in your spiritual preparation.

You are led into a inner sanctum of sorts. It is the most beautiful room you have ever seen or experienced in your life. The sunlight is penetrating down, down through the inside and that sun hits upon the center of the room where there is a beautiful, warm fountain. You proceed forward to this fountain and you notice that the water that is coming forth from this place is warm and colored....beautiful golden, white, and amethyst colors misting very lightly on your body as you step through it every part of you is cleansed and washed in the vibrant colors and water of this fountain. On the other side of this fountain is a beautiful lotus blossom floating in the water that sustains this fountain. You know that your place is in the middle of this lotus blossom. You realize instinctively that the purpose of this blossom is to heal every part of your body. It is to heal the physical, the mental, the emotional, and the spiritual aspects that make up you.

You sit down in the middle of this beautiful lotus blossom and the minute you sit down you are energized by a universal life force energy that you start to draw up from your Root Chakra. As you draw the red from your Root Chakra you draw it up, mixing with the orange that is the Sacral Chakra; as this chakra opens and vibrates, it draws up, up to the yellow that is the Solar Plexus chakra. As that center vibrates and opens, it draws the yellow up, up to the green that is the emerald of the Heart Chakra. Then your Heart Chakra vibrates, vibrates and opens and draws up, up to your Throat Chakra. The beautiful blue of your Throat Chakra vibrates and opens and draws up to the Pineal, the Third Eye center...the beautiful indigo (blue-violet). As it vibrates and opens up, up to the violet of the spiritual, Crown Chakra, you feel the warmth from your root up, up through all of these open, vibrating chakras...up through the crown; then flowing out the top of the crown. You are showered in all these beautiful vibrant colors of your chakras. They are vibrating and showering your entire body with the healing warmth of the water from that lotus blossom, that healing blossom that is drawing up, up through your body washing you and any problems, cares and old patterns away. You feel the warmth, warmth of that shower and your body is being born anew.

You open your hands and you place them on the side of your Crown Chakra and you feel the warmth of your hands aiding in this healing process and you bring your hands down from the Crown to the Third Eye. You place your fingers over the Third Eye area, your palms over your eyes, and you feel the warmth of your hands aiding in the healing process. Then you bring your hands down to your Throat Chakra, placing your hands over your throat, fingers together, you feel the warmth of your hands aiding in the healing process. Then you bring your hands down to your Heart Chakra, placing one hand above the other on your upper chest, and you feel this warmth, this healing warmth penetrate your Heart Chakra...clarifying and opening, and healing your heart. Then place your hands just above your navel on your Solar Plexus; feel the warmth from your hands aiding in this healing process. Move your hands just below your navel, you feel yourself warming and healing your entire abdomen with this healing process. Then you place your hands on each side of your hips at the place where you are sitting and you feel your Root Chakra; feel it with the warmth from your hands, aiding in this self healing process. Then bring your hands back to your heart and your Heart Chakra and acknowledge that every part of your body has been energized by the universal life force energy. As you acknowledge that this is so, you will remember this experience whenever it is necessary for you to do so. In your mind's eye you step forth out of the lotus blossom center, back through the healing shower of the fountain, and every part of you is glowing with the fresh vibrant feeling of new life, and new life force energy that has entered your body.

As you step back through the fountain, you realize that the warmth of the sun that is shining in through the cathedral ceiling has dried every part of you. Your special guide reaches forth and hands you a beautiful white healing robe that you wrap around yourself and tie at the waist. You have a great love and a great gratitude for all those that are here and present at this time. You begin to hug each and everyone that has come to help you with process to guide your forward from this time on in the spiritual path. You acknowledge that it is time to leave this special place. You are aware that you may return here at any time. You follow forth toward the door out. As you reach the door, another guide steps forth and hands you a gift. You examine the gift and then you acknowledge the gift with great gratitude and love. It is for you to use in your healing work.

When you are ready, you step forward out of the doorway to this great city, out into the cosmos once again, coming back to the place where you were before. You descend down, down a starry, celestial stairway. You feel warm, fresh, new, better than ever, better than before. Every cell, every nerve, every muscle, every part of your body has been washed with the light of the universal life force energy.

You are grateful for this opportunity, and as you draw in a long, deep breath, you realize with a bit of sadness that the time has come to return to your own reality...time to return to the here and the now. You begin to notice that you are feeling your fingers and toes, feeling your body return to the room where you are now, clear headed and peaceful. Shanti.

MEDITATION
For
HEALING THE CELLS IN THE BODY

In your mind it's a beautiful warm, spring day in the mountains. All around you are signs of new life and new beginnings. You see the fresh, vibrant green grass and the trees with new leaves. You hear the sound of moving water. Just ahead in the distance is a beautiful waterfall that cascades gently into a shallow, still lake. As you get closer to this waterfall, you are able to see that the waterfall is made of millions of drops of beautiful, healing, blue water. You wade in the quiet, shallow pool of water until you are directly beneath this gentle waterfall. Feel how soft and cool this healing, blue water is. Feel each and every drop as it begins to flow through your hair and across the top of your head. The healing color of blue is so vibrant that you draw it deep inside of you. Guide it down, down, down, until it reaches and opens your Heart Center. Feel this cool, healing, blue color as it enters your bloodstream with every beat of your heart. It flows throughout your body nurturing every cell, every nerve, every fiber of your being. The blue color is cleansing, calming, cooling, and healing every cell throughout your body. Feel it as it is flowing through you now. It relaxes and releases tension in your body. The muscles of your shoulders relax. Your arms to your fingertips relax. Your back relaxes and releases any tension. The middle of your body relaxes, and your legs relax. This radiant, blue, healing light is now flowing down through your stomach, relaxing and healing all of the organs in your middle body. Your internal organs are touched by this healing blue light: your stomach, liver, spleen, kidneys, even your intestines and bladder are soothed and healed by this blue light. Feel your lungs relax as you inhale peace deep into your respiratory system.

Now you see this blue light penetrating the DNA and the RNA of each and every cell of your body. Feel it as it is cleaning and refreshing every cell; healing every cell from the inside out. It is making each cell well, healthy and whole; well, healthy and whole. Your cells have all that they need to be well, healthy, and whole. Complete. You are now one with the color blue of the still, healing lake. You are as placid, calm and peaceful as the lake. Allow the healing to flow through you and around you. Allow the blue, healing color to nurture you. Allow yourself to be a calm, cool, healing drop in the placid, blue lake. You are one with the lake, you are well, healthy, whole, and complete. You are one with the lake, flowing down, cleansing every cell. See every cell as new, healthy, well and whole. Each and every time that you say the color blue, see the color blue, or hear the word "blue," your body responds with a healing power and initiative. Blue is healing. Your body and its healing power recognize the word "blue," as a signal to heal. And it is so because you and your mind ordain your cells to be healthy, well, and whole.

You hear your own innervoice as it speaks these words:

"If there are any cells that exist in my body that are not now all complete, healthy, well and whole, I ordain my body to wash them out through the healing waters of the lake; flush them out through my system so that they can be released and disposed of properly. Transmute, and release these cells. Only healthy, well, and whole cells exist in this body. I love, respect, and heal my body. I am a vessel for healthy cells, cells that nurture my body and make it well and free of disease. I live in harmony with the universe. All of my cells respond to my voice as I intend for them all, each and every one of them to be healthy, well and whole. Ten times ten, my cells are healthy, well, whole and complete. And it is so because I ordain it. I am a child of the universe, I deserve to be healthy. My cells are healthy, I am healthy. Every day in every way I am manifesting great health and happiness in my life. I am healthy, I am happy, I am whole. Each and every time that I see or sense the color blue, I am healed. I embrace my health. I enjoy my health. I am worthy of health. I claim health for my body. And it is so." (Note: Read on tape to listen to for at least 30 days.)

"The fresh and beautiful moon is traveling in the utmost empty sky. When the mind-rivers of living beings are free that image of the beautiful moon will reflect in each of us."

Chinese poem

MIND RIVERS:
THE POWER OF REIKI

by
Master Karyn Mitchell

Knowing all I know of Reiki now,
I honor its great gift in my humble life.
Abundance in Health and Happiness flow to me
Like a radiant, warm river of brilliant crystal.
Loving all allows us to gratefully share this Divine Gift
With those who desire to be free mind-rivers of healing.

Free your mind. Free your heart. Free your spirit.
As you hold this glorious gift in the palm of each hand,
You are the creator of your own universe, you are Chiron,
The once wounded healer, now transformed and limitless.
It is so. It has been ordained by you, the creator-healer
 The dreamer of perfection incarnate, living in harmony.
You who reflect in your radiant, loving, healing heart
The lifeblood of the star-filled Cosmos: of All That Is...
You, the Divine Gift, reflect the wondrous image
        of the
            beautiful
                moon.

OTHER REIKI BOOKS BY KARYN MITCHELL

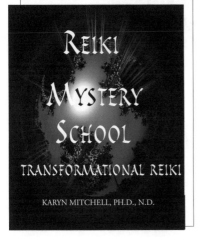

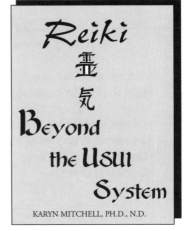

Transformational Reiki™ Spiritual Healing Secrets including: Youthing; "Kotama," The Power of the Word; "Unisonium," Achieving a Higher Vibration; Reiki Iro (color); Meditations; and Other Mysteries. Healing Applications for Specific Diseases.
ISBN # 0-9640822-5-X
Retail price $19.98

Advanced techniques in Reiki healing practice. Reiki treatments for AIDS, Cancer, & Pregnancy. Introducing "Trans-Reiki™," Infinity Healing, the Interdimensional Chakras and Bodies & Yin-Yang Reiki. Transformational Meditations and Chakra Affirmations.
ISBN # 0-9640822-2-5
Retail price $19.96

Also by Dr. Mitchell: **Walk-Ins/Soul Exchange**
ISBN 0-9640822-4-1 Retail $17.95
The Sacred Truth/The Bloodline of Sophia
ISBN # 0-964082-9-2 Retail $18.95

Guided Meditation Tapes by Karyn K. Mitchell
Order 815-732-7150   mitchell@essex1.com $10 each pp in U.S.

- Experience Reiki
- Absentee Healing & Self Healing
- Meditation for Spiritual Advancement
- Soul Star Meditation/Soul Beyond The River
- Journey to The 9th Chakra/Moving Into Light
- Finding your Soul's Purpose
- Depossession as Therapy
- The Emerald, The Eagle, The River & You
- Find Your Spirit Guides   • Healing Your Past
- Past-Life Regression as Therapy
- Cancer and Chemotherapy (Self Hypnosis)
- Meeting Your Ancestors •The Gift

- What is Reiki? & Reiki Meditation
- Healing the Cells of the Body
- Healing the Child Within
- Weight Reduction
- Smoking Cessation
- Soul Retrieval
- Gentle Depossession
- Asthma
- Past Life Relationships
- Abductions: How, When & Why?
- Healing Bridge
- Self Hypnosis/Feng Shui the Spirit

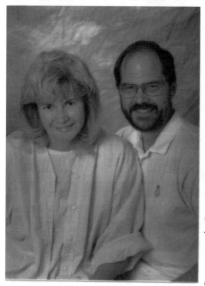

Karyn K. Mitchell Ph.D., N.D., R.M.T., C.Ht.
Biography

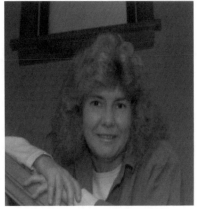

Karyn Mitchell is a Naturopathic Doctor with a Ph.D in Psychology. She is an international teacher and speaker in the fields of Reiki, Hypnotherapy, Vegetarian Lifestyle, Meditation, Natural Medicine, and Shamanism. She has been a student of Psychology, Metaphysics, Religion, and Philosophy for over twenty-seven years. She is a member of the American Naturopathic Medical Association, and is registered with the Minnesota Naturopathic Association. She has taken the Five Mindfulness Trainings with Master Thich Nhat Hanh, a Buddhist Monk ordained in the Zen tradition. Also, Karyn is a graduate of the Silva Method, and has studied Shamanism with Michael Harner and Sandra Ingerman (The Foundation for Shamanic Studies). She has studied other cultural dimensions of shamanism in other countries and from other instructors. She is a medical intuitive and mystic dedicated to sharing the spirit of compassion and love for people, animals, plants, and minerals.

She is a Holistic Counselor, and a Certified Reiki Master-Teacher of the Usui Shiki Ryoho School of Reiki. She is certified through the American Board of Hypnotherapy as an Instructor of Metaphysical Hypnotherapy, and is an instructor certified by the International Medical Dental Hypnotherapy Association (I.M.D.H.A.), and the American Association of Behavioral Therapists. Karyn holds further certification from the National Association for Transpersonal Psychology in the areas of Clinical Hypnotherapy, Transpersonal Therapy, Analytical Hypnotherapy, and Past Life Regression Therapy. She and her husband, Steven Mitchell have co-founded A.R.T., the Association for Regression Therapists, and "Reiki Path" School of Reiki Instruction. They have both dedicated their life's work to assisting others with their spiritual growth. Karyn maintains an office at Haven Holistic Center in St. Charles, Illinois and works as a Holistic Counselor, Naturopath, Reiki Practitioner, Teacher, and Regression Therapist. Her personal spiritual philosophy is to guide students and clients to a place of personal awareness and empowerment.

Her books, <u>REIKI A TORCH IN DAYLIGHT</u>, <u>REIKI BEYOND THE USUI SYSTEM</u>, <u>REIKI MYSTERY SCHOOL</u>, <u>WALK-INS/SOUL EXCHANGE</u>, and <u>SACRED TRUTH/THE BLOODLINE OF SOPHIA</u> published by Mind Rivers, are available at most book stores.

Reiki Mystery School™ Class offerings: The mystery teachings that transcend this book; the mysteries that we share in a class that are too sacred for any book.

CLASS DAY ONE: TRANSFORMATIONAL REIKI ™

This class is for the serious aspirant of the Reiki Path, and the prerequisite is Reiki Level II. We share the secrets of Reiki as a healing art. The ancient roots of Reiki are revealed to assist in the dynamic process of healing and spiritual growth. Rites related to enlightenment, immortality, and rejuvenation are offered. We study the Tibetan perspective of disease as related to karmic actions. The Ancient Tibetan Fire Attunement that links the Soul to Interdimensional Reality and Soul's Purpose is offered. This increases the vibrational rate and healing empowerment within the individual. In this class, you are introduced to color healing and the Interdimensional Chakra System and Interdimensional Bodies that activate deeper healing in the physical body. You learn of a healing field called the Unisonium, where practitioner and healee meet to create a more intense energy potential for healing. Meditations in class include: Meeting your Interdimensional Guide; Interdimensional Chakras; Planes of Existence; Soul's Purpose; and melting into the Unisonium. This day focuses upon increasing student empowerment.

CLASS DAY TWO: KOTAMA: THE WORD ™

Kotama is the application of Sacred Sound. We use sacred Mantras and seven powerful scripts to assist in healing each of the seven Bodies: Physical, Mental, Emotional, Spiritual, Light, Cosmic, and Interdimensional.

Advanced Healing Techniques for self and others will be an integral part of the Kotama Teachings. Such techniques include specific hand placements to activate a pulse in the Meridian System that opens a gateway to each of the seven Bodies. This pathway encourages deeper healing and release of old patterns that exist from this and other lifetimes as related to karma and disease. Four ancient symbols are shared including the symbols for manifesting, increasing energy, compassion, and a symbol to disperse negative energies in yourself and others. You receive the Tibetan Mandala of Protection. This day focuses upon utilizing your increased power to help others heal more effectively.